# Learning to Walk Again

# Learning to Walk Again

◆

## How Guillain Barre Taught Me to Walk a Different Path

*Ann K. Brandt*

Writer's Showcase
New York  Lincoln  Shanghai

# Learning to Walk Again
## How Guillain Barre Taught Me to Walk a Different Path

Writer's Showcase
an imprint of iUniverse, Inc.

For information address:
iUniverse, Inc.
2021 Pine Lake Road, Suite 100
Lincoln, NE 68512
www.iuniverse.com

ISBN: 0-595-25823-9 (pbk)
ISBN: 0-595-65360-X (cloth)

Printed in the United States of America

To George, my husband, coach, and cheerleader

And to Sally, my mentor

...God turned to good what was meant for evil.

—Genesis 50:20

# Contents

# 1

# GBS (Guillain-Barre' Syndrome): The Mystery Disease

"Theresa passed away." The voice on the other end of the line had brought me in from the crispness of a late fall afternoon. My husband was outdoors moving the ladder, preparing to paint the next section of upstairs window trim. I was supposed to be There, holding on and hoping he wouldn't fall and crush us both. Into the pleasant rhythm of our lives had entered death. And illness—again.

Shaking, I stepped outside. "George, remember that patient I visited last week? She's dead!" Together, we stood silently, mourning a woman I had seen only once. "Her poor husband. George, you should have seen how worried he was that day in ICU."

Nobody is supposed to die from Guillain Barre. I didn't. Some don't survive with everything they had before the illness. But it's not supposed to be a fatal disease. It was for Theresa who, just when she was getting over the worse part, had aspirated something from her feeding tube into her lungs. Our little Guillain Barre support group was collectively aghast. *There but for the grace of God go I* was, I'm sure, thought or uttered by more than one patient or caregiver.

Theresa's husband had been so concerned when he called me. She was still in intensive care, he said, but he was sure I would be allowed in to see her. Would I visit? GBS had hit her hard and fast. Within twenty-four hours her entire body was paralyzed, including her eyelids. She was trapped in her body. Her husband had been dividing his time

1

between the hospital and the Internet, researching everything he could find on GBS. "They had to suture her eyelids shut," he told me. When I saw him standing beside her, gently stroking her hand I thought I had never seen such a gentle and loving caregiver.

Caregiver is an endearing term given—or earned—by the spouse or significant other who is often left to struggle with uncertainty and upheaval, worrying all the while about the outcome of this strange illness that attacks often in minutes or hours, sometimes in days or weeks. When I was sick, George, like many others, was not prepared to be a caregiver, but he learned fast. I had always been in charge of household chores and George had been the main breadwinner.

Suddenly, he found himself in a crash course learning to do laundry, grocery shopping, and food preparation. The folks at our local super-market took him under their wing and he proved to be a quick study, especially in the meat department. I would come home weeks later to a full larder. When I was released from the hospital for the recovery phase he was almost overwhelmed to find himself in complete charge of a patient who could not walk and who required large amounts of medication at regular intervals. Moreover, I moaned a lot. The sudden-ness of the disease had caught him by surprise, and our lives spun out of control in those first weeks.

Few people know enough about Guillain Barre Syndrome to recog-nize it during that first crucial time when it is destroying the protective coating around the peripheral nerves, making fingers and toes numb and tingly, then generating complete or partial paralysis. Worse yet, many general physicians have not had enough experience or exposure to GBS during their training and first years of practice. Without a neu-rologist, often precious time is wasted until a correct diagnosis is obtained. The pain that is often present in GBS is rarely recognized as part of the disease, but many people I've talked to remember pain as a significant part of their GBS experience.

What is GBS, where does it come from, whom does it attack, and how does it affect our lives? Most of all, why do some patients emerge intact from the experience while others spend the rest of their lives in wheelchairs? Many things about GBS still need answers.

The biggest question is how do we go on with our lives once we have been declared recovered. The assurance that we'll get it all back rings hollow with many GBS survivors. How do we cope with an experience that has attacked our bodies and left them compromised in some degree? Even if we learn to walk again on our own, our bodies have suffered an assault that changes us forever. This need not be a negative; in my case GBS has evolved into some positive events. I like to think that a sense of humor, a strong will, curiosity, and faith in God all played a big part in my recovery and my journey down a different path.

When I emerged from my haze of pain and paralysis and began to put my life back together I wanted to know more about what I had just been through. Many books have been written about other neurological diseases, but library and bookstore shelves are bare in the category of Guillain Barre Syndrome. Save for Joseph Heller's account of being hospitalized and Sue Baier's horrifying story in *Bed Number Ten*, written in 1985, I could find nothing written for the layperson.

My meeting with reality came in the form of GBS patients, some in recovery for years. I met most of them at the first Guillain Barre Syndrome Foundation International symposium I attended. There I was shocked to find many former patients still in wheelchairs, many still using walkers. Of those still mobile, I noticed crooked fingers, stiff limbs, halting gait. I heard horror stories of ventilators and intensive care units. Many had suffered through a series of misdiagnosis before GBS was recognized as the cause of numbness and tingling. Many, like myself, had experienced a serious fall before diagnosis. I listened with a growing sense of awe and humbleness.

Two things have become quite clear in my mind regarding Guillain Barre. There needs to be a greater awareness of this disease (syndrome) in the medical community so that patients presenting with both typical and atypical symptoms can be tested and diagnosed without undue delay. The other thing is that no one case of GBS appears to be the same. Very few cases seem to follow a precise pattern of developing symptoms or even of recovery.

Once a correct diagnosis was made and we knew what the problem was I considered myself lucky. I was only partially paralyzed and have no memory of being on life support or experiencing near death. I was walking with a cane after six months and now walk on my own.

This disease has taken me down a path I never expected to walk. I've talked to people I never expected to meet and done things I never expected to do. I've learned to walk again with a different purpose.

# 2

## *Influenza Season and Flu Shots*

Sixty-five people looked on while Jean pinned the gardenia on my lapel. "Thank you," she said, "for volunteering to be Denver's liaison. And thank you for getting this together." Then, I heard applause. *How did I get to this point?* I smiled in the direction of the four people on the committee who had helped me get ready for this day. My husband George stood by the door, beaming proudly.

I had never dreamed of conducting a symposium for anything, let alone organizing a support group or visiting hospital patients. Not until after I had recovered from Guillain Barre Syndrome did I realize what it's like to be sick and helpless. I had been so healthy all my life; even delivering four children into the world had been relatively easy. Life had been so uncomplicated, ordinary days and unremarkable chores, until I came down with GBS. In the long days of recovery, I found myself with a new title: survivor. It is human to inquire of God why we suffer, and why we survive. Even though it may not be evident at the time of our trials. I'm convinced that whatever we suffer, God is there to help us endure. When we survive, God is there to show us what to do next. At that moment God was there to help me conquer my fear of public speaking.

I cleared my throat. "Thank you for coming. Welcome to the first annual Colorado Guillain Barre symposium."

During the rest of the meeting my mind drifted back to that December day in 1996 when I sat at my kitchen table grading papers. Many times I had said to my colleagues at the college that English teachers should receive extra pay. I would watch teachers of other disciplines put their test results into a machine, press a button and presto, out would come the grades. Or so it seemed. English teachers, on the other hand, had to read each essay carefully and use subjective judgement to decide a grade. Students couldn't argue with a machine, but they often argued with their English teachers.

On top of that, the end of the semester occurs just when a person wants to be starting Christmas preparations instead of rushing to get last minute papers and exams graded. Every year this happens, I would grumble to myself. . Why do these kids still keep making the same mistakes on their papers.

I was grumbling that afternoon in December. *Why do my shoulders ache so?* Annoyed, I reached to massage my neck and shoulders. How tired a person gets just sitting hunched over all these hours. I needed a change, a bit of exercise. Swallowing one last drop of tepid coffee, I stood up and called out to George. He was in his workshop in the garage, building a computer for one of his customers, "I'm going out for a walk. Not taking Lucky. I'll be back in an hour or so." Our big dog would want to do the walk her way: run, stop, sniff, start up again. I was in no mood for interruptions. I wanted to walk steadily and briskly. I had to work the kinks out of my back and shoulders.

I covered the distance around my neighborhood with long swinging strides. The fresh air was bracing and it felt good to be released from prolonged sitting. I've never been happy sitting in one spot for long periods. Moving along, I reflected on how much sickness there had been in Denver that fall.

"Half the students were absent today, and three teachers in the Department called in sick," I reported to George one afternoon. George and I had both been battling one cold and cough after another since we had our flu shots in October. Instead of keeping us well, the inoculations had seemed to bring on more sickness. We had prided ourselves on staying free of colds and flu, but this year had certainly been an exception. George had even suffered such bronchitis that he had given up smoking after forty years of heavy use. One Sunday in the middle of the church service, he sat down suddenly. . "Drive me home," he whispered. Startled, I looked down. His face had a bluish tinge. *A heart attack!* Without a word, I got him into the car and sped home.

Fortunately, we keep a canister of oxygen on hand to help with migraine and cluster headaches. A few puffs and George's normal color returned and he breathed easy again. What a scare! That was the last day he smoked a cigarette after forty years of smoking. Our post flu shot troubles did bring about one good thing.

In the midst of all the illnesses, Front Range Community College had been in some state of remodeling ever since I had come to work there in 1993. That semester work crews were ripping apart the section of the building where my classroom was. The heating system had run amuck and the whole building was affected. The classroom was raging hot and my office was freezing cold. No amount of chicken soup and vitamins had been able to keep me healthy that season. Students never get enough sleep and seem to be in a perpetual state of stress, and this year they were falling ill in even greater numbers. I could have sworn that one morning I saw germs hovering in the air just above one young man who sat huddled in his seat, shivering in spite of his heavy coat and wool hat. Coughing, sneezing and dozing, the students and I looked at each other with glazed eyes and struggled on.

I turned a final corner and headed home from my walk. One more week and final exams would be upon us. As soon as I turn in my grades I can begin Christmas preparations, I thought. Then George and I can get ready for the long awaited holiday visit in California with some of our children and grandchildren. But first things first, I reminded myself. A pile of essays still waited to be graded. We all have to get through this time somehow.

# 3

## *Shots, The First Symptom*

I returned home from my walk, improved in mood but not in body. That worrisome ache was still there. No kinks had been worked out. That night was our turn to help serve dinner to men at a homeless shelter with some friends from our church. When we had cleaned up and left, our appetite led us to our favorite spaghetti restaurant. There, conversation flowed around me while I allowed myself to relax for the first time in weeks. What had brought me to this point of overwork; I had added one too many things—one too many commitments, a small voice answered. *You know what you shouldn't have committed to.*

What greed will do: In August someone from the Colorado Department of Education had called with an assignment. Would I research and write one hundred annotations for a new literacy project. This work would be in addition to the teaching load I had already signed up for. As I was forming the words for a refusal, I heard "and we are prepared to pay...." That was all I needed. Now here I was over committed worse than I had ever been. The deadline for finishing the work was drawing near and anxiety about finishing on time was giving me chest pains at night.

All too soon our relaxing evening was over and it was time to go. My legs cramped when we stood up to leave. Strange, I thought, but legs do that sometimes when one has been sitting for a long time. Walking to the car, I felt weak and achy. *Am I getting sick again?* I had just begun to recover from the last bout of fever and coughing. "Wait for me!" I called out as the others strode ahead. My normal brisk pace had disappeared. I probably overdid that afternoon, walking so hard and long.

There was never enough time for regular exercise. *How out of shape you are*, I chided myself. .

Returning home, I looked at the two big roasting pans crusted with dried spaghetti sauce. Bits of pasta clung to the sides, and the big serving spoon lay on the bottom of one—a repulsive sight. "We'll just soak it for now," George said, reading my thoughts. I was too tired to do anything but fall into bed and drift into an exhausted stupor until just after midnight.

Then it hit—pain so severe that I felt my body was ripping apart. Careful not to wake George I slipped out of bed and crept upstairs to the living room. Maybe if I could just sit quietly on the sofa and look out the window at the sleeping neighborhood it would take my mind off whatever is wrong with my back and legs. The pain seemed more intense on the right side. What did I do to myself? Had I slept the night before in an awkward position? Did I twist my back carrying my heavy briefcase? I waited for the Tylenol to take effect so I could go downstairs and get back to sleep. I had only one class to teach on Thursday, I thought, so the next day wouldn't be too difficult. Toward morning I staggered back to bed and dozed for a couple of hours.

"You don't look so good. Why don't you call in sick." George took the coffeepot out of my shaking hand and finished measuring out the grounds.

"No. Remember that Front Range doesn't pay if you take off a day. I can do this."

"OK, stubborn."

Somehow I drove myself to the college. *Damn, wouldn't you know, no parking places close.* The pain dragged at me when I tried to pick up the pace from office to classroom. Arriving a few minutes late, I propped myself against the desk and announced that I was sick. The students remained in their seats. "Go, really go. No class today."

They looked at me as if suspecting a trick. I had never canceled class before. I nodded and the exodus began. Within one minute the room was empty and I was free to go home.

The next night was worse. At 2:00am I knew with a sinking heart that I would need more relief than what a Tylenol or aspirin could give. A thousand evil fingers were pressing into my lower back and all the way down my hip and thigh on the right side. Years before I had been caught off guard by a brief experience with sciatica, but a muscle relaxant had soon put me back in shape. So I took one of George's muscle relaxant pills. It did nothing.

I couldn't take another night of pain. And not only was the whole miserable business interfering with my well planned schedule, it was downright agony. I wanted to conquer the pain once and for all. I woke up George. "I think maybe we should go to the emergency room." George was only half asleep anyway and he readily agreed. He wanted to get this problem out of the way as much as I did. Whatever I had done to my back was having dire consequences.

So we drove off into the night. The world at 2:00am in the Denver suburbs is very quiet. Few lights shone in windows. Traffic was all but nonexistent. The emergency room of our little local hospital was almost deserted. George answered insurance questions, filled out forms, showed his IBM medical coverage card and I described the pain.

Pain is such a nebulous thing. When doctors ask patients about their levels of pain on a scale of one to ten, what would be a three for one person might be a ten for someone else. And vice versa. But that night no one questioned my pain. I didn't know it then, but that call for pain relief would be the first entry on an unofficial indictment of my mental balance.

I have always been a private person, used to keeping my troubles to myself, confiding only in my husband or children. That night I was ashamed to be complaining of something so inconsequential as a back-ache. I was even tempted to turn back and return to the car. But the morphine came with a stick of a needle and with it blessed relief. I knew nothing but a gentle blackness. I have heard how people can become addicted to morphine and now I can see why. It seems so easy to erase one's troubles with a quick stick of a needle. After I rested for a while George half carried me back to the car.

The next day I decided to take a proactive approach. I was still relaxed from the narcotic and from the temporary relief from pain. So I called up our acupuncturist in Boulder. She had helped George and I in the past with various problems. She could see me just before noon, and I drove up to Boulder with high hopes for complete relief and an end to all that inconvenient suffering. I was more than ready to take up my normal course of life once again.

Harriet looked doubtful when I tried to describe the source of the pain. Once again, as the day progressed so was the pain progressing. My short respite and sense of relaxation had disappeared. But Harriet used her magic touch and I experienced some relief. On the way home, though, the pain began to return and by the time I walked in the door I was miserable once again. *What muscle has pulled? What tendon has stretched?* I cried with frustration.

George came home from servicing a customer. "Call Dr. Jones," he suggested. "This is Friday. You can't go all weekend like this.

Doctor's appointment secretary managed to squeeze us into his schedule and we drove off anticipating a quick fix, figuring that we would just lay the problem at the feet of the doctor and all would be well. By suppertime we had the diagnosis: stress. At that time stress seemed like an easy thing to deal with. I was forgetting the baggage of pain that came with that effortless diagnosis. But stress could be put away until there was time to deal with it. Anything else would be too time consuming, too complicated. I was so sure that the Valium and the painkillers would serve as a magic bullet. With high hopes I hurried to have the prescriptions filled.

# 4

## *Stress as an Easy Answer*

"Valium! I feel like a kook," I complained. "And these pills don't even work." The only other time I had taken Valium was to dull the pain of having my last baby. *How can this pain be worse than labor pain? And why does it always creep up on me at night?* It was like a crouching tiger getting ready to spring. And the attack launched again the following night, Saturday. The painkiller didn't work either. I tried the heating pad, the ice bag. Sitting, standing, or lying down: there was no position remotely comfortable. "How can you sleep like that?" I muttered, looking at George peacefully unaware of my suffering. People who sleep were in a different world from mine at that moment.

I hated to wake George again. He has never been a good steady sleeper and waking him up with my moaning and groaning wasn't helping. George had his own problems with a history of two neck fusions and carpal tunnel surgeries with complications. Jumping up out of bed and driving around in the middle of the night is never anyone's favorite thing to do. But I remembered what relief I got from that shot of morphine two nights before. "George," I whispered. "Wake up. Maybe if you just rub my back." But it did no good. We set off for the emergency room.

The folks at the hospital were not pleased to see us again. A group of white coated figures seemed to converge on me. I sensed a feeling of disapproval. No more morphine, but I could have Demerol. These people looked serious as they conferred with each other. Frowning, one of them addressed George. "We're going to admit her."

"Fine." George wanted to get a diagnosis, some reason for this mysterious pain and plan a program to fix the problem. IBM had paid him for many years to be a problem solver, a reliability engineer, figuring out answers to countless perplexing situations. He was convinced that there was an answer to this puzzle. But I was beyond caring, riding the downslide of the emotional roller coaster I would be on for the next couple of weeks.

That night the thin hospital mattress covered with a rubber sheet that seemed to crackle at my every movement drove me to standing up and walking from bed to window in a fruitless effort to get away from the pain. A blizzard had come up and the highway three floors below had few cars. Most drivers were safe at home. I didn't feel safe and I wasn't at home. How I wished for my old life, the ordinary rushed routine I had grumbled about just last week. *What did I do to make this happen?* If I could just figure out what it was all the suffering would come to an end and life would get back to normal.

George arrived late the next morning. "The roads are bad. I passed two accidents on the highway."

I didn't want to hear news outside my problems and my sense of humor, so handy in many situations, had deserted me. "We're supposed to be in California in two weeks." Our plans were going off track. Then I voiced the unspoken. "What if we can't go?"

George said nothing. The look on his face told the answer.

"But, our plane tickets are bought and paid for."

Still George said nothing. He's not a big talker when he's worried or trying to analyze something. We had planned our Christmas holidays around a trip to California to visit our son George. Diana, our daughter-in-law was expecting their first child. Our oldest daughter Kathy and her husband Scott and their two boys Brett and Shane would fly out from Tucson. Our youngest daughter Alice with her husband Willie and their son Thaddaeus would come down from Seattle. It would be a wonderful family reunion and as our Christmas present to the grandchildren we were all planning to go to Disneyland on Christmas Day. Then we would spend the New Year back in Colorado with our second oldest daughter Cindy, her husband Charlie and sons Carson and Crosby.

Instead, the family was in turmoil. No one thought I would live through this unknown malady. Lucky for me that I didn't realize their concerns at the time. I also didn't think to feel sorry for my doctor in his fruitless efforts to identify the source of my pain. Years later, I imagine the feeling of failure a conscientious physician must suffer when he or she cannot locate the source of a problem.

With any disease in the diagnostic stage, the relationship between patient and physician hangs in the balance. The patient wants answers, fast. The physician works under pressure. If he or she jumps to hasty conclusions, the results can be disastrous. On the other hand, if diagnosis is not nearing, the patient and family become uneasy. Tension results. Patients bear some responsibility here and should be willing to seek a second opinion. Most doctors will not be offended if you ask to bring in a specialist. However, I was not only acting as the passive (in pain) patient, but I was actually assisting in my own misdiagnosis by describing my recent heavy work, indicating anxiety over deadlines, and emphasizing how stressed I had been feeling. Little wonder that my doctor jumped in with the idea of stress.

Stress seems to be the buzzword of contemporary living. I have heard others tell of being diagnosed with stress in a hard to pinpoint disease or syndrome. Doctors seem to use the term as a last resort. In more facetious moments I wonder if there isn't a separate class in medical school on the malady of stress. Stress is a word that is tossed around with impunity by the media and the general public. "Stressed out" is even sometimes thought of as a mark of success. Is it any wonder that we think of any kind of pressure as stressful. But, while stress does compromise the immune system it shouldn't be considered the primary cause of any illness.

I had always been strong physically, emotionally and spiritually—or so I thought. When my oldest daughter went into labor with her first child I was there to reassure her that labor wasn't that bad and that all four of my deliveries were like a walk on the beach. (I may have overplayed the easy part somewhat.) But I had survived illness, surgery, and adversity and come through with aplomb. Until now. Now we were up against something with no name, no immediate cure, and it was getting worse. Talk about being out of control! *Just take it away, God!* Whatever plan He had for me, I wasn't buying it at that time. I just kept crying.

Worse than the pain and uncertainty was the unspoken message from the medical community I was perceiving, that it was all in my head. Since that time I have heard of other women's physical complaints being brushed aside by medical professionals. Stress, they tell a patient, anxiety. Certainly a patient becomes anxious when the source of pain and discomfort remains a mystery. The suffering intensifies, the patient complains, and the doctor is even more convinced that the cause of the problems lies in the mind of the patient. It becomes a vicious circle. One woman, suffering with the pain of Guillain Barre onset was actually hospitalized in a psychiatric hospital. I faced each encounter with my doctor with a mixture of guilt and anger. *Am I imagining all this pain? I'm not crazy if that's what you think.*

I come from a generation that still thinks of doctors as some kind of magicians who can look at a person and discern what is wrong. *You're the doctor. Fix me.* This attitude isn't fair to anyone. It certainly doesn't work in the case of a rare disease. Worse, this childlike demanding faith can block essential communication between doctor and patient.

Most patients, by the time they arrive at the emergency room or hospital admitting office, are extremely sick and have no knowledgeable advocate. With no clear thinking person working on the problem everything falls squarely on the physician. Much more is expected of doctors today as we explore scientific advances and learn to use the tools that technology brings.

What's more, it isn't enough that doctors be technically competent; now we expect them to be compassionate, patient, perceptive listeners.

Some insurance companies have restrictions and regulations governing how much time a doctor can spend with a patient. It's a rather frustrating situation all the way around. I don't know what is to be done about the direction in which our present health care system is heading, but it's something I ponder now that my own crisis is past. Open and honest communication is a must in one of the most important relationships of our lives and it's being so overlooked in so many cases.

Caregivers, otherwise known as the worried family member, significant other, or hired professional, need attention also. Our GBS support group meetings always include some portion where patients and caregivers divide into separate groups for casual discussion. The first time we did this I had a sense that these discussions were much needed. I asked George for his opinion.

"I wish I'd had someone to talk to like that when you were sick," he said. "It would have been so much easier." Always a problem solver, this mystery pain was one problem that he couldn't solve. His nerves were becoming frazzled from frustration and from lack of sleep. It couldn't have been much fun to have keep dragging me to ER and listening to my tale of woe.

He needed information and he wasn't getting it. He needed reassurance that this scenario wouldn't keep playing out forever. And he needed rest and relief from his own physical problems. Many support groups, I have since discovered, pay special attention to caregivers. Sometimes I think that in their own ways, caregivers go through more discomfort and mental agony than the patients.

I, on the other hand, thought only of finishing my obligations and carrying out our holiday plans, ignoring how out of control life had become. I had long since given up on finding the root of the problem. Just get rid of this pain and everything will be all right, I reasoned. On some level, also, I was blaming myself for letting things come to this. What I could have done differently, I could not fathom, but it must have been something. Naturally as I became more anxious and worn down, my body tightened up and the pain exacerbated. Pain builds on pain.

Doctor Jones was becoming frustrated. He had ordered MRIs, Xrays, and blood tests, only to come up with no discernable reason for my pain, then the increasing clumsiness. December is not a good time to fall ill with anything not clear-cut or easily diagnosed. Doctors go on vacations and leave colleagues on call for them. In the second week of my ordeal I was left at the mercy of an on-call doctor who was clearly annoyed with me.

When my pastor came to the hospital to give me communion, I saw Dr. Herd start to hurry into the room, then stop short. *Thank God for professional ethics. He has to wait.* I imagined Dr. Herd pacing up and down in the hall because seconds after Pastor Brad left, the doctor appeared for a one minute visit. I had the feeling that he wished I would just go away.

It never occurred to me or to George to go to another hospital or try a different doctor. One's doctor was one's first and only choice. Strengthening that attitude was the fact that there was no neurologist on staff of that small hospital. It was a fine new facility; all the rooms were private and the staff was nurturing and caring when I had my hysterectomy there three years before. There was none of the rushed atmosphere sometimes present in big city hospitals. But I realize now that expertise in rare diseases can be limited in smaller hospitals and this lack of specialized care can lead to horrific events.

# 5

## *Not MS But What?*

That night in the hospital was the first of many on a roller coaster of hope and hopelessness as test after test proved inconclusive. After a few days Dr. Jones came to my room after another round of tests. "Well," he said, with a sigh, "we don't know what you have, but you don't have Multiple Sclerosis." I found myself actually feeling disappointed in that announcement. My feet had taken to slapping on the floor in a type of waddling gait I had noticed on two people I knew who had MS. I was ready to settle for MS just to relieve the suspense. At that point I would have gladly settled for something concrete—something definite. I would have been able to accept, adjust and go on with my life rather than continue in a state of limbo. Whenever I hear of people not getting a definitive diagnosis and dragging on for years not knowing what is wrong or how to fix it, my heart goes out to them. A disability is bad enough but once one knows what it is, lifestyle can be accommodated. With my usual blind optimism I thought, *I could have done MS.* A person has to be pretty desperate to have such thoughts.

Although I was sedated for most of the trips through the MRI and CAT scan machines so that the infamous thump-thump sound was not bothersome, I'll never forget the blood collector. Little glass tubes rattled on the metal tray as a figure dressed in a plain blue cotton uniform entered. "This won't hurt," he murmured, wrapping a rubber cord around my arm just below the elbow. *Not much.* The word hurt had taken on a whole new meaning in the larger scope of things. He didn't seem to be satisfied with one tube of blood. I lost count but eventually he took his leave, rattling down the hall to his next victim.

I recall that someone came with a little gadget to put on my thumb, measuring my oxygen intake. A pulse-ox, they called it. I was tempted to retort that I don't usually breathe out of my thumb, but then thought that these folks must know what they're doing. Also, I was learning that many medical people are not alert to jokes, at least while they're working.

Another figure in a plain blue cotton uniform padded softly into the room. "We're going to Xray." *OK. They'll look at my bones and find something that can be fixed. I'll go along with that.* As if I had a choice. Off I went on the big gurney ride down to Xray. By then I was feeling a bit foolish about all this fuss. It was getting to be embarrassing. We were all at an impasse. Evidently I was the mystery patient. It's so inconvenient to have mysteries around just before Christmas. The only thing worse than pain was embarrassment and despair. "Take me home," I pleaded with George. Not knowing what else to do, he asked the doctor for a discharge order.

The next day I mentioned the possibility of a strained back muscle to George. He seized on the idea and off we went to the chiropractor. Our friend Terri had recommended Dr. Waters who had an office nearby. If he can't fix you, he'll tell you so," she assured me. This will be my chance to be fixed, I thought with confidence. George and I approached the entrance to his office with high hopes. I had never been to a chiropractor, never thought it necessary. I had always thought of chiropractors as practitioners a bit outside the pale of normal medical practice. Once they got their hands on you it was a lifetime commitment to regular visits of twisting and pulling. I had heard many people speak of visits to the chiropractor for "adjustments." It never sounded like anything I'd be interested in doing. But I was desperate. *If Terri says this guy is OK it must be so.* I was open to anything. How quickly one's views can change.

This man came highly recommended by others as well. He had corrected many problems. I ignored the part where Terri had spoken of his forthright manner. He *would* fix me. It would happen because I wanted it to happen. He would just lecture about poor posture and strained muscles, maybe give me a little chart showing correct ergonomic positions at the computer, twist some magic spot in my back and all would be well.

We were ushered into the examining room immediately. Dr. Waters took each foot in his hands. My confidence grew. "Twist this way. Now turn down. Then up. Let's see you walk." I obliged. "I don't know what you have," he concluded. But it doesn't involve muscles or joints. I wish I could help you but I just don't know." My hopes, so high a moment before, fell with a thud. Another dead end. George helped me limp out to the car. Walking was becoming painful and difficult. We looked at each other. "At least he was honest," George said, starting the car and staring straight ahead.

"Yes, but now what do we do? Where do we go? There were no answers. George was silent and we drove home lost in our own thoughts. It was becoming clear that I needed a specialist, but what kind of specialist? Our experience with medical emergencies was limited to OB GYN care for me; even so you couldn't call one miscarriage, four deliveries and a hysterectomy emergencies. George had been seen by various neurologists through the years with his intermittent bouts with cluster headaches. Looking back, I realize that our knowledge of neurologists should have given us the sense to call upon one of them. But we didn't take the initiative to go outside my current sphere of care. The disappointment with the chiropractor had sapped our energy.

One big barrier for primary care physicians in diagnosing rare diseases is medical training. Medical schools don't seem to devote much time to training in recognizing seemingly disassociated symptoms. GBS is not the only thing that has been incorrectly diagnosed or undiagnosed. One hears horror stories of people almost dying before getting proper care. Fortunately, I was not about to die, and we have come a long way in the last century of patient care. But the sad truth is that the emphasis on research and on training medical students seems to be on the tried and true, the publicized diseases that bring in money for research and for which donations are easily solicited. Doctors themselves are frustrated over this state of affairs.

To add to our discouragement the pain grew worse and the next day I became a reluctant hospital patient again. The next day, Tuesday, would be final exam day for my students at the college and I wouldn't be there. Who could I trust with my students? George, dear patient George. "How would you like to go to my classes tomorrow and give the exam? It's all written and on my desk at home," I asked.

He grinned. "Sure."

It turned out that the students loved him. He gave them as much time as they needed to complete their essays and told them he didn't want them to become stressed as he was seeing first hand what stress can do. (It seemed everyone was buying into the stress theory for want of anything else.) Later I enjoyed reading all the little notes of appreciation and encouragement that students wrote at the bottom of their papers.

Meanwhile, all of our children must have been conferring with each other and with various sources as they found them. Kathy, our oldest daughter, telephoned me from her home in Tucson and we chatted about a lady she knew who had a similar pain that was never diagnosed and had continued for fifteen years and counting. Her malady was considered chronic. How cheery. I was not reassured. Our second oldest daughter Cindy was using her home computer from her home in Colorado's high country to research various diseases.

Our son George had been preparing to have us all visit him and his wife Diana in California. Our sixth grandchild was due to arrive in April and we were pretty excited about having a granddaughter. We had purchased our plane tickets several months before. Hope was fading fast that I would be well enough to celebrate anything anywhere let alone take a long trip.

Alice, the youngest was busy researching in her own way from her home in Seattle. One of her neighbors was a neurologist and, talking with him, she prepared a list of questions that we should be asking. We should see a neurologist, she emphasized. But who? Where does one find a neurologist seemingly out of nowhere? We had not yet realized our rights as health care consumers. We didn't know to ask for a referral, let alone who to go to for such information. Worse, we hadn't faced the fact that we have a responsibility to demand proper care and a correct and timely diagnosis.

# 6

## *Lady, You need Psychotherapy!*

Stubbornly, or stupidly, we stayed with our primary care physician and stubbornly, he pressed on with tests that proved nothing. I was becoming weaker and sicker and the tests were becoming an endurance contest. Communication between doctor and nurses must have been breaking down, as I was soon to find out.

One morning the breakfast cart lumbered up the hall, dishes rattling, and institutional cooking smells wafting through the air. *When is my tray coming?* Hospital food is better than starving to death. I pressed the bedside button. There had to be some oversight here.

"No food or drink this morning." Bright flowers on the nurse's smock belied her grim message. "You're having an MRI."

"What?" I've had MRIs before and didn't have to fast for them."

"Susie!" called Flowered Smock over her shoulder. "She's having an MRI. Can she eat?" There was then a hushed conversation out in the hall followed by long moments of silence and isolation while I waited for Flowered Smock to get the word. Finally, a cheerful presence entered my room bearing a tray with a nice tasty bowl of corn flakes and a cup of cold coffee. It took the place of lunch. Another piece of information to store in my medical information bank: The kitchen and the unit staff are sadly out of touch with each other.

By the second week of in and out hospital stays and countless tests, some of them almost as painful as the original pain, we took Dr. Jones aside for some serious conversation. "We have to get a neurologist in here even if there aren't any on staff," George said.

23

Dr Jones frowned, pondering. Then he brightened. "We'll call Dr. Smith," he said. As he left the room to make the call, I turned to George. "Isn't that the doctor who didn't help you with your cluster headaches?" George nodded. The seeds of doubt were there but sometimes desperation makes a person travel a dark path.

Dr. Jones came back from his phone call, smiling. "Dr. Smith will be here tomorrow afternoon and we'll take her over to the clinic." *Take who over to what clinic?* I didn't like the sound of this.

Sure enough, the next day, with a nameless feeling of dread, I got dressed slowly and awkwardly. Shoes and socks were impossible. I couldn't lean forward without falling over and my hands were not working right. I felt like a child while George tied my shoes. After signing me out for a few hours, George drove me to the clinic. As the car pulled up beside the building my feeling of dread took on new proportions. *This was it. I remember.* "Don't you remember, George how he charged you for pain management and nothing helped. He wanted to give you all that medicine that you'd already tried years ago? This is that same place."

Too late. We were ushered into an examining room where Dr. Smith and another white coat clad man were waiting. *Who is that? Now what?* Good afternoon, Ann. *Grr. I hate it when people are so casual about first names when I don't even know them.* And how are you today? "Fine," I said. I actually said fine.

"Let's see how you walk," ordered Dr. Smith.

I must have looked amazed. *Walk? Buddy are you a dreamer.*

Dr. Smith turned to George. "If you'll just wait outside." George obediently stepped outside. How obliging were we going to be. "OK, Now just hold on to my arm here." Tentatively I slid my backside forward to the edge of the examining table and tried to stretch my toes downward. "That's it, just stand up." Both men caught me as I began to pitch forward. "You're doing very well." *What?*

George was summoned back into the room. "Let's go into my office," said smiling Dr. Smith. Somewhere in the back of my mind I was remembering the story of Red Riding Hood when the wolf called her into grandmother's cottage. Dr. White Coat had disappeared. There was a thirty minute discussion on the subject of stress and pain during which my mind began to wander. I caught up just in time to hear Dr. Smith say, "And we should begin psychotherapy today."

I was led away into Dr. White Coat's office. George was removed to the waiting room.

After an hour of discussing stress with Dr. White Coat (at least I now knew his position in the clinic), I was about overdosed on the subject of stress and was ready to return to the hospital and lie down on the nice black rubber mattress with the thin cotton sheet and rest my weary and pain-filled body. Thankfully, it turned out that George also had been wary and had refused to sign the contract that would in essence give the clinic a blank check. Months later he refused to pay the bill when it arrived and we never heard from those folks again. I wanted a real neurologist. But it was not to be for a while.

# 7

## *Tender Mercies of Nurse Torture*

Being sick messes up a person's mind. I have forgotten the worst parts of that ghastly time before diagnosis, but one day especially stands out as a short journey into hell—The Day of the Tests.

By that time I had lived through MRIs of the lumbar and sacrum areas of the spine and had begun to rely on a catheter most of the time to empty my bladder. So when the day began with an announcement that once again I was not to have breakfast, it was too much. "Why? I inquired.

"You're scheduled for an MRI this morning." A tired looking nurse unwrapped the blood pressure cuff and scribbled something on a chart. *Here we go again.* Ignoring my look of distress she looked over the top of my head and launched into an account of how she dreaded working through the day. It turned out she had been fighting a losing battle against a terrible cold.

Her companion paused, bedpan balanced under her arm, nodding sympathetically. "Yes, I had a fever last week and even had to miss a day of work. I can't afford to miss any more pay." A lengthy conversation went on involving cold germs and epidemics while I prayed for no one to breathe on me.

Then I had a thought. "I am hypoglycemic and hypothyroid. I haven't had my Synthroid in a long time, and why do I have to fast for an MRI." Frustration poured into my words.

Nurse Cold Germ looked surprised and left the room to come back within minutes. "You can't have anything to eat or drink. You're scheduled for surgery later today." *Surgery? Now they're going to have to cut me open to find out what's wrong?* I didn't like the sound of that. Worse yet, dinner the previous evening would have to sustain me the whole day. *My last meal.*

By afternoon I lay on a hard table in the downstairs day surgery room awaiting the hospital stomach expert. There really is such a thing as "esophagoastroduodenoscopy." Reading my records months later, I was impressed. But right then George and I were playing the waiting game. Dr. Expert was two hours late. In no time, I was under anesthetic, or maybe I fainted from hunger. I'm told that a little camera was inserted into my stomach, I was sent through the CAT scan machine, and was given an epidural. Such efficiency: When the patient is unconscious, might as well make good use of the time, I always say.

The epidural was supposed to kill pain. It did the opposite. Epidurals deliver narcotics and local anesthetics directly to the spinal nerves. Guillain Barre pain comes from demylinating peripheral nerves. The protective coating around the nerve (axon) is being eaten away by attacking antibodies and leaving an exposed nerve. Just as when insulation around our outdoor telephone cable wears away it results in static on our telephone line. I just wish I had known all of these details at the time I was going through the ordeal. A simple explanation might have made it easier to bear. Anxiety elevates pain levels. On top of the epidural being ineffective, it actually added more discomfort in the small of my back.

*Am I being a sissy? A complainer?* Having four babies and a miscarriage within ten years had not been this much of an ordeal. I thought back to when my youngest daughter Alice was born. George had come home from work and I met him at the door. "How far apart are your pains?"

"Two minutes. Do you want a sandwich before we leave?"

"Two Mintes! Get in the car."

Turned out he was right to be in a rush. We got to the hospital with thirty minutes to spare. So it had been with baby number two, Cindy. Baby number one, Kathy, had been a bit more reluctant to make an appearance and baby number three, our son George, was born three weeks after my mother had died suddenly. He was early and I was not in good shape. Overall, though, I had a pretty good record of delivering babies efficiently and without a lot of fuss.

I hate making a fuss. I'm also not used to people treating me as if I'm a bother. So the night nurse in recovery and I did not get along at all. "Why are you breathing like that?" Was I breathing with the pain or gasping because I couldn't get air? A little of both, I suspect.

Another nurse came over to my bed and inquired if I had ever tried meditation. I didn't have the strength to retort. Starvation had added to pain. Irrationally I wanted to run away from the pain and was caught in the act of trying to raise myself up. "Enough of that." I couldn't believe she was tying me to the bed.

"What happens when I need to go to the bathroom?"

She hesitated a moment. "Let me know and I'll help you."

Somehow this promise was not very comforting. *If she thinks I'm a bother now what will she say when I'll be ringing for help all night.* The catheter had not become a permanent fix at that time. I wanted to call George and have him come and rescue me from this person I perceived as a sadist. But Nurse Torture put the telephone out of my reach.

It was the worst night of my life. At 6:00am I inched my way to the head of the bed and stretched to reach the cord. Nurse Torture was not in sight. I pulled the phone to me and called George. "Come and get me." Then I fainted.

Soon I felt the familiar callused hand in mine. "Rough night?"

"That nurse. She tied me to the bed and wouldn't let me use the phone." I was sobbing with relief.

George saw Nurse Torture standing in the doorway. "That one, huh? I'll be back in a minute."

I heard his voice but couldn't make out the words. After a while I heard the cart with breakfast trays rattling down the hall. My tray had very little on it: a cup of lukewarm coffee, a small box of dry cereal, and a small container of milk. I was too weak to reach for the tray.

"That's all you get?" George had returned. He started for the door again.

"Please stay. I'm not even sure I can eat this. What did you say to that nurse?"

George's face tightened. "I don't think you'll have any more trouble with her."

Thankfully I never saw her again.

# 8

## *Narcotic Overdose*

During all of this fuss and confusion about what was or wasn't wrong with me, something happened to reveal why hospitals and medical personnel are so suspicious about bruises and bumps on incoming patients.

When in frustration and anger, George brought me home and away from the tender ministrations of Nurse Torture, I was amazed to find how much trouble I had getting out of the car. It seemed to take forever to get my legs to move. It was December 14, ten days since the mysterious pain had first struck. *May be this weakness is just from lack of sleep,* I thought. George had gone on ahead, happy and confident that now I was home and all would be well.

There I sat, half in and half out of the car, my feet dangling like bowling balls on the ends of strings of cooked spaghetti. They didn't seem to be getting any messages from my brain. Finally, hanging on to the open car door, I lifted myself out and staggered toward the house in a swerving pattern. *I must look like I'm drunk. I hope no one is looking.* Tripping over the door jamb, banging and crashing against the doorway and the furniture, I finally entered the house, annoyed with my feet, myself, George, and the world in general. "What's wrong? Where were you?" George looked surprised that I had lagged behind.

I could only glare. "I've got to sit down."

That night I chose the upstairs guest bedroom and George took a sleeping pill for a good night's rest in our bedroom.

The next part of that night is fuzzy. After the usual sleeplessness I took some of the pills prescribed by the three different doctors who had seen me. They had all accumulated on the kitchen countertop, and I was too tired to notice how many there were of what. The next thing I remember is hearing a violent crashing sound that seemed to go on and on. Then the back of my head hurt and I was annoyed to find myself sprawled face up on the downstairs hall floor. *Damn!*

George came rushing upstairs. "What the hell happened!" It was not a question. I remember the sensation of being stuffed into a coat and half carried to the car. We were off again to the same hospital we had vowed never to go near again. It seemed that I was doomed to keep returning like a bad penny.

The admitting staff in ER must have been regarding me with suspicion by then because records show that they gave me a shot of Narcan, the standard response to drug overdose. Those words "Narcotic Overdose" are actually written in my hospital record, much to my chagrin. Also in that record is a report that I had been seeing a pain management specialist, referring no doubt to the session with Dr. White Coat at that clinic.

The serious young men with the clipboards and nametags didn't seem to have much of a sense of humor. When asked who the President was I responded with what I thought was a lighthearted remark. "Don't you read the papers?" That earned me a bad mark. "Pt is belligerent." George tried to intervene in my behalf, earning him a bad mark. "Pt's husband is controlling," reads the report. So much for humor and helpfulness. I was once again trundled off to the inpatient floor. It was all getting a bit old.

That evening I took a little stroll with a walker the unit nurse had thoughtfully provided. In the hall I promptly tripped over my robe in full view of a group of nurses and visitors. A smartly dressed young man rushed to my aid. "Are you all right?"

Trying to maintain my dignity I clung to the walker, hoping it wouldn't wheel out from under me again. "I'm fine," I mumbled and made as hasty an exit as was possible under the circumstances. I must have made quite an impression because a couple of years later when I visited a sick friend at the same hospital, one of the nurses on the floor remembered me as the patient in the long red robe. I knew which robe she was talking about—the one that tripped me when I tried to take a drink of water at the drinking fountain. Who wants to be that famous.

During that period it seemed that nurses had begun to take an inordinate interest in my home life. It became tiresome to keep answering questions about anyone hitting me recently. I have since discovered that hospitals are bound by law to investigate when bruises as visible as mine are found on incoming patients. The whole back side of my body was one big bruise from going bumpity bump down a whole flight of stairs like a limp rag doll.

Beds with rails, nurses to take me to the bathroom—it was all bad enough but Christmas was coming and the hospital was beginning to empty of patients. To add a touch of grim irony, several groups of carolers swept through the halls, but they didn't cheer me up. People don't want to be in hospital at Christmas time unless it's an emergency. Was I an emergency? I certainly was a mess.

# 9

## *Diagnosis: Guillain Barre*

A real neurologist is coming! Those welcome words were received with a mixture of joy, relief and cynicism. A part of me was saying *Yeah, right.* Another part was saying *Finally! Praise God!*

It turned out that the second part was right.

I had been on the prayer list at our church for two weeks and on the prayer list of churches of all our friends and family. Pastor Brad had given me communion my first Sunday in the hospital. He and his wife had visited, bringing a poinsettia plant and best wishes from the whole congregation. George was beginning to accumulate a nice collection of baked goods brought over by neighbors concerned he would maybe starve in my absence. The prayers had been for healing, but that wasn't happening just yet. What we really needed, George decided was a correct diagnosis. So he and Pastor Brad prayed. God heard and responded.

"Please," we said to Dr. Jones, could we have a real neurologist, not that other one, but a real one."

Dr Jones looked doubtful. "Well there is Dr. Raymond but he's not on staff here. I've never met him but he comes in to consult once in a while."

"Call him now." George was in no mood for further discussion on the matter.

In the short time it took to confirm that indeed Dr. Raymond would be there that afternoon to examine me we almost held our breath. All our hopes were pinned on the arrival of Dr. Raymond. It was a long morning. I thought back to the evening before when the

Christmas carolers had trooped through the almost empty unit, trying to spread holiday cheer to staff and patients. What a mockery it seemed to have red and green decorations at the nurses' station and in the hall. I thought of the child George and I had seen in one of the rooms. The parents sat silently by his bed. He lay so still. To this day I think of that child and wonder what happened to him. The room was empty the next day.

Dr. Raymond arrived, serious and unsmiling. No jokes, no small talk, he took my feet in his hands. "Turn your foot this way." I looked at my foot in astonishment. It wouldn't move. "Bend it upward please." Nothing. *Are these my feet?* I wondered also why he was looking at my feet when it was my back that hurt. But instinctively I trusted him. He was gentle and kind. After tapping on my knees and getting no knee jerk response he stood up. ."There are two tests I'll need to run yet to be sure, but it looks like acute inflammatory demyelinating neuropathy—Guillain Barre"

A memory of something I had read years ago flashed in my head. "It's a polio kind of thing isn't it?" I also remembered that the person in the magazine article had been sick a long time.

"Yes," he nodded. "But you'll get it all back."

I put that statement in the back of my mind to think about later. "Can I go back to work next month? Spring semester begins in three weeks."

"No not next semester," he said beginning to turn away. "I'll order those tests and we should know by the end of tomorrow if it's GBS for sure. Meanwhile I'll order Neurontin to help with the pain."

I lay back in the bed exhausted and pleased. At last we had something to work with. Before the supper trays were delivered that night the blood collector came again, rattling his little glass tubes in the metal tray. But this time he was on orders from Dr. Raymond. That night after taking the new medication I slept for three wonderful uninterrupted hours, the first restful sleep in over two weeks. Until then I had been sleeping in snatches of fifteen to twenty minutes at a time. So

I considered Neurontin the super drug although it affects everyone differently. It is one of a family of anti seizure medications and was fairly new on the market at that time. Some people become hyper on Neurontin, others are seemingly unaffected. Now on the rare occasions that I need pain relief even a small dose will make me feel fuzzy.

The next day, right on schedule, Dr. Raymond came to administer the spinal tap. I had heard horrible stories about spinal taps: the pain, the headache afterward. But my worst fears didn't come to pass.

"There'll be some discomfort but I'll try to get this over with as quickly as possible," he said, slipping on latex gloves. He turned to the unit nurse standing beside him. "Alicia, can you help me here?"

The procedure was over in a few moments. If there is a good technique for gentle spinal taps, Dr. Raymond had that technique. We had made another step in progress. Elevated protein level in the spinal fluid is usually the defining moment in diagnosing GBS. The next day, to confirm what the spinal tap had revealed, Dr. Raymond ran an electromyograph, a nerve conduction test (NVC). Now there was no doubt; it was GBS.

After giving thanks for prayer answered, a definitive diagnosis, we faced a second problem. Who would treat me and where? Where do we go from here? In the following months we would learn the importance of prompt, correct physical therapy so necessary for effective rehabilitation. Range of motion exercises are usually begun when patients are still in hospital. In the worst cases of paralysis the therapist starts by gently massaging the patient's hands and feet, then progressing to raising his arms and legs slowly, increasing the range gradually. Muscle atrophy sets in quickly and it does no good to delay movement. Here is where professionals must be careful to neither overdo or underdo rehab treatment. Many patients go directly into a rehabilitation center for a period of time, then take rehab as outpatients, preferably in a facility with a heated therapy pool on the premises. Patients who exercise in a heated pool with specially designed equipment and under the supervision of trained professionals do very well in recovering strength without fatigue and pain.

Dr. Raymond had left orders that I was to be released to residential rehabilitation. He had been called in for what is known as a consult. That meant his job was done and it was time to follow through on the next step. He came in to say goodbye and Merry Christmas before he left for the holidays. The hospital by then was on skeleton staff and patient rooms were mostly empty. What a hollow, lost and lonely feeling. Worse yet, the rehab center that had been recommended wouldn't take me as I had a psychiatric record, a result of my meeting with Dr. White Coat. With no other options apparent, George took me home. It was the day before Christmas Eve.

# 10

## *All Alone*

I was in a bad spot. No doctor, no hospital, a disease that no one seemed to know how to treat, and all the doctors we knew of were off on vacation. George wanted advice. I just wanted to go to sleep and wake up when it was all over.

So problem solver George got on the phone in an effort to get information on what one does in our peculiar circumstance. First he called our good friend Terri, a retired RN, and she came over to care for me.

When Terri walked in the door, I knew I would be OK even though I couldn't manage stairs and had no appetite. "You should eat," she said, looking authoritative. "How about some soup?"

I nodded. Soup sounded as good or bad as anything else.

Terri stayed most of the day, making sure I rested and ate. It was Christmas Eve and she had her own family to care for and her own Christmas to get ready for, but she was one of many friends who would come to our aid in the months ahead. We would have plenty of emotional and physical support that I will never forget. From the time I was diagnosed, except for those scary hours before I was finally admitted to our big city hospital, the feeling never left that everything would be all right. I was in God's hands and it felt good.

One very special person in our church congregation is an experienced registered nurse, serving at that time as Ethics and Human Values chairperson in one of Denver's largest hospitals. When George called Anna for advice she assured him that it is not out of line to terminate a doctor-patient relationship if it is not working. George had done so when he took me out of the little hospital this last time. It took courage but it was the right thing.

We now think of Anna as one of a series of angels on earth sent to help us through a maze we didn't even know existed, let alone know how to navigate. After recovering from GBS I took the time to read a book that Anna recommended: *Honest Medicine* by Dr. Donald Murphy. Dr. Murphy suggests healthy skepticism when evaluating your relationship with a physician.

Since GBS I have often reflected on what we learned during that period of bouncing around, seeking proper care. Patients and physicians have an obligation to each other. The doctor must call in a colleague for consultation if he or she can't find a cause for symptoms. It's unfair to revert to weighing psychological causes against physical symptoms. And the patient has a responsibility to insist on proper care. This is not always easy.

One must have an advocate—someone who can deal with decision making while keeping a clear head. Sickness often strikes without warning, so it's a good idea to talk about the issue of emergency health care ahead of time with your spouse, close relative or friend. However, someone too emotionally tied into the patient can become pulled into panic and confusion. George had to consciously choose to detach himself emotionally for the time it took to get me out of my bad spot that Christmas Eve.

Fortunately, we had good insurance. Many hospitals and clinics can become uncooperative when they find themselves dealing with uninsured or underinsured. Managed care and other situations that prevent long term relationships with health care providers pose a real obstacle to doctor-patient partnerships. When family members are working to communicate with the health care providers and the physician listens and communicates effectively, you have the best of all worlds.

Unfortunately, doctors can have valid reasons to be skittish in our litigious climate. It's important to remember that doctors are real people.

Since recovery I often play the "what-if" tape in my head. What if I had been one those rare patients who doesn't survive GBS? What if the nerves leading to my breathing muscles had been paralyzed and diagnosis wasn't prompt enough? What if I hadn't complained of pain? What if I had just tried to tough it out without seeing a doctor. Maybe I hadn't been such a weakling after all. Maybe pain had saved my life.

George experienced an unnerving conversation with a chance acquaintance that he didn't reveal until I was well into recovery. Someone's elderly mother had suddenly lost strength in her legs, then her whole body became weak and she had difficulty breathing. By the time she saw a doctor, it was too late. She died. What if I would have passed away, leaving George with a burden of paperwork and unmade decisions? Worse yet, what if something had gone wrong and I were permanently dependent on life support? These thoughts made me realize the temporal aspects of everyday life—how we are wrong to think that we always have tomorrow to communicate with our friends and family, to organize our lives, to decide how we want to be remembered. We hate to think of these things, but everyone is going to die some day and unpleasant as it is, we need to plan while we can think clearly.

It was brought out after my recovery that while a DNR (do not resuscitate) order is a matter of individual choice, the time to make that choice is before the emergency. By the time the patient is intubated (put on life support) the next decision to be made is whether or not to remove life support (pull the plug). This leaves your friends and family with some difficult if not illegal choices. Equally important, though, is a medical durable power of attorney which assigns decision-making powers in all medical situations to someone you choose. These are personal issues, relating only to you and to those close to you, but important to everyone who uses the health care system in some way.

One lesson that we learned during that time of limbo between hospitals, during the most unimaginable time to be sick, was that once you have left one institution the way I did you are not fresh material for a second facility and will be viewed with a bit of suspicion. Doctors and hospitals are wary of patients who appear to be jumping from one situation to another, seemingly looking for a diagnosis that fits their needs. This is not to be confused with people seeking a legitimate second opinion. George now admits that he was scared when he signed the waiver for that hospital to release me, not knowing what the next step would be. To be fair, hospitals need to protect themselves against patients suing for anything that occurs as a result of leaving without authorization.

The only possible way I would be admitted as a patient in a new hospital would be through the emergency room. Even that would not be easy. I had been promised a home health nurse and even as I had heard the words I had thought my skeptic thought again. Even so, I put off even thinking about any hospital. I just wanted to sit next to George and draw comfort from being at home. We had no decorations, no Christmas tree, no family. It was George and I against the world. And our faithful dog Lucky. So we sat, too tired, too beaten down to make any decisions.

# 11

## *Christmas Eve and Off to the Hospital*

There is something about the calming presence of a dog or cat and the act of stroking its soft fur that can make one's present troubles melt away. As George and I sat in the living room like two defeated soldiers returned home, my thoughts drifted back to the strange way this dog had come to be ours.

The year before, Lucky had appeared on our doorstep as a lady of the streets, just past being a puppy but with a lot of puppy playfulness. She wore no collar and no identification and seemed pretty determined to have us as her owners. We always tell people that she picked us out. At the time, however, she was a diamond in the rough. She had a habit of peeing wherever she happened to be, indoors or outdoors. Sofas, chairs and beds were doggy trampolines and pillows were for tossing and dragging around. She never chewed anything and that was probably her redeeming feature. That and her sweet personality.

It was obvious that she had been abused because the command to come brought out a strong flight response. In the presence of visitors to our home she would either run to another part of the house or stand between George or me and the other person. Often I was reminded of the song *Lean On Me....* Sometimes she would almost knock us over with leaning. I don't think she had ever been on a leash until the day I took her out for the first time. Off we went, lurching down the street with me grasping at fence posts and street signs to keep my balance.

41

And that was *before* Guillain Barre when I still had my strength and stamina.

By the time we had Lucky a year, she had been through two rounds of obedience school and had begun to form a strong bond with George and me. That bond was strengthened forever during the unstable days of my illness. George took her with him whenever he went to the hospital or when he did errands. She waited patiently in the car endless hours until he would come to walk her or pour her a drink of water from a little thermos he found for her at a flea market. (One of George's ways to relax when under stress is to shop. He did a lot of shopping in December 1996.) Lucky was a moral support to me during recovery at home. Dogs are so straightforward: no pretending, no false cheer, just a soft nuzzle and a quiet presence. I don't know if it was the gravity of the situation or coincidence but that dog calmed down a lot as soon as I got sick.

And so the "three Musketeers" as we called ourselves by that point, sat listening to Christmas music when the doorbell rang. It was the home health nurse. My cynicism had been unfounded after all. The nurse looked at me. "You belong in a hospital." *Tell me about it.* "Where's your phone?"

A lengthy conversation went on in the kitchen between the nurse and whoever she was talking to on the phone. George and I sat silently, occasionally hearing the words Guillain Barre. The person on the other end of the line didn't seem to be giving any answers to her questions. Presently she hung up. "They'll call back."

I was in desperate need of a catheter, nauseous, bloated and miserable. My feet felt like they were encased in heavy socks and the pain in my back had become a part of me. There was not a drop of energy in me. To put us at ease while we waited, Miss Winters began to chat about the big swine flu epidemic of years before and all of the Guillain Barre cases that came about as a result of the flu vaccine. "We had people on cots in the hall waiting for a room—all Guillain Barre." When I told her about my flu shot and where it was given, she grimaced. "That company had a bad batch this year." My present bladder shut down is part of the disease, she told me.

When the phone rang, her conversation was short. We were to go to the ER at University. I would be admitted that night. *Praise God!*

Praying that she was right, we drove though streets brightly decorated for Christmas. Inside, families were together opening gifts or getting ready for late night Christmas Eve church services. I wondered what our family was doing in California at that moment.

# 12

## *A Two-Minute Christmas*

The car pulled up in front of the emergency room entrance. This big city hospital was a lot different than the small community hospital I had been running back and forth to all month. A grim faced security officer guarded the metal detector at the door and the waiting room was empty save for a tired looking man and woman dressed in worn coats. Yesterday's newspapers were strewn about the dimly lit room. We were called into the triage room almost immediately. *When do I get to pee?*

The inevitable question came; "How are you?"

For once I told the truth. "Terrible. I feel like I'm going to die any minute."

What a relief when I was settled into a cubicle and hooked up to a Foley catheter. Shortly, Julie, the RN in charge took a urine sample for lab testing and brought me some iced cranberry juice. She didn't look surprised when she returned to report that I had a roaring bladder infection. "Do you want some more cranberry juice?" Soon I was drinking and peeing pretty steadily. I hadn't realized how thirsty I'd been.

Then began the procession of doctors and neurological tests. "Touch your fingers together—-Touch your nose—Push against my arm." I was beginning to anticipate all the commands. It later dawned on me that in a teaching hospital everybody wants to get in on the action. GBS is rare and this may have been a golden opportunity for some of these young residents and interns to see a disease they may not see again until they are in private or public practice.

Some patients don't care for teaching hospitals; they feel it violates their privacy. My view is that teaching hospitals have seen a wider variety of diseases and symptoms than private hospitals, thus broadening the areas of expertise available. Large teaching hospitals also have a large network of contacts to consult. If the hospital staff reaches an impasse in diagnosis, it will quickly research until the problem is solved. This big city hospital was housed in an old building but its ideas and knowledge were state of the art. I felt better emotionally than I had in weeks.

Except for pain. The pain was getting worse and lying on a gurney in the emergency room wasn't helping my back. By the time the Admissions representative had taken more information from me and advised me to send my watch and purse home with George, it was three o'clock in the morning. I saw how exhausted George looked. "Why don't you go home now and get some sleep. I'll be all right."

His small moment of hesitation told me I said the right thing. "Are you sure?"

"Yes. Go."

Then I was alone with the knowledge that I would spend Christmas in a hospital. Baking, shopping, decorating—those activities existed far out of my present world, no longer matters of importance. Miles away the children and grandchildren were having Christmas without George and me. It didn't matter. Nothing mattered anymore. My resistance had been worn down to the point I was trembling as an orderly rolled the gurney past a lot of white walls and into an elevator. *Would we ever get to a room?*

The ward was nighttime quiet and dimly lit. Two nurses wearing Santa hats were watching a Christmas concert on television. Music played softly in the hushed atmosphere. It was 4:00am—Christmas morning. The nurses set to work settling me in bed, taking my vital signs with a formidable looking device that made what seemed an intolerable grinding sound, like a pneumatic drill. That sound would become part of my daily routine. "Something for pain, please." I was close to tears.

The nurse patted my hand. "Soon dear. We have to wait for the order to come up here."

So I waited. Time seemed to stand still while I saw behind my closed eyelids orange and red monsters and shooting flames. I tried to imagine cool green pastures and still waters, but the orange flames won. *This is my punishment for always concentrating on so many silly preparations instead of thinking why we really have Christmas.* My Christian background had always given me Christmas but over the years I had grown accustomed to keeping Christian holidays without giving much thought to their meaning. There is nothing like a feeling of complete helplessness to bring on a session of self-examination.

My thoughts were interrupted by the arrival of pain pills and more water and cranberry juice. I couldn't seem to get enough liquid. Then I lay back and tried to be still, willing the medication to take effect. I turned my head slowly toward the window and saw the morning star, bright and steady as it much have been for the wise men following its direction to the manger in Bethlehem two thousand years ago. Never had the lessons of my Sunday School days been so real. A gentle peace came over me and the pain slipped away. Knowing that Jesus knew my suffering and would help me heal was my Christmas comfort. Before falling asleep I whispered, "Happy Birthday Jesus."

# 13

## *A Lost Day*

When I woke from a short troubled sleep that first day in University Hospital, I realized with a sinking feeling that it was Christmas morning. My first impulse was to call George. It took a long time to reach the bedside telephone. After five or six rings, he answered, sounding far away and weak.

"Is that you? Are you OK?" Why do we always assume that everyone at home is just fine when in fact family members are stressed and worried. I thought of when I had given birth to our first child over forty years before after two false alarm trips to the hospital. By the time we went for the real thing George had been quite frazzled. On the surface he always looks calm, but underneath he comes apart in shreds. He must have been very shredded that day. "Were you sleeping?"

"No." In that one word he sounded like a little lost boy. No, he couldn't summon the energy to drive up to Longmont.

"But won't you be lonesome? What will you have for dinner?" Our friends Sandy and Don had invited him over for dinner so he wouldn't be alone for Christmas. How good it is to have caring friends. "You should go. All I'm doing is sleeping."

"That's OK. I'll be all right." He didn't sound all right but I was too tired to hold the telephone any longer. Months later, reflecting on that period of time, I concluded that a close loved one may not be the best patient advocate. It's too hard for one person to be supportive mentally, emotionally, and physically. One person cannot be at the patient's side, keeping things going at home, keeping track of information on the disease and procedures, and communicating with doctors.

Something eventually has to give. Support people, sometimes referred to as caregivers, are in danger of burnout.

Someone a bit more emotionally removed could keep track of procedures and medications for future reference, keeping a clear head without becoming frazzled. Not all patients want to know complete details of their illness but some people have questions and they should be answered. Luckily Kathy, our oldest daughter, was due to arrive the following week. Scott had volunteered to watch their boys and keep the household going while she would be in Colorado. I will be forever grateful to Kathy for providing a steady influence on George and giving me emotional support in the hospital.

I dozed most of the day. The room, designed for two patients, seemed empty. The door looked like it was a million miles away and I was in the middle of a large space, such a different feeling from the night before. Everything looked white. What was wrong with me? I wished that someone would talk to me. And I felt cold, chilled to the bone. The nurse had given me an extra blanket that morning but I couldn't stay warm. I have since discovered that other GBS patients have had this same distorted awareness of surroundings and sensations. Some people have experienced frightening hallucinations. Our internal thermostats seem to go out of business as well. Sue Baier, author of *Bed Number Ten* tells of not being able to cool off. It seems to be a part of this strange and frightening disease.

George sounded anxious when he called and we talked a second time. He had not recalled anyone telling him about Guillain Barre, what to expect, what causes it. He remembered our flu shots in October and how sick we both had been all fall and winter. He couldn't forget how I had coughed so hard and so long that we both thought I had whooping cough. Once more we remembered how his bronchitis had become so bad that he couldn't breathe and he gave up smoking. After forty years of heavy smoking, he actually gave it up—with the help of the nicotine patch. And now he was home alone on Christmas Day, frightened and without cigarettes for comfort.

Sometime during the day, the door opened and two white-coated figures walked in. "I'm Dr. Widrow and this is Ellen a student here at the University." Ellen nodded and smiled. I felt sorry for her having to see patients on Christmas. Looking back, I imagine she was feeling sorry for me. There is, after all, not a major rush of business on Christmas Day, even in hospitals. There followed another neurological test with the touch your nose, bend your foot routine. This was getting rather old. All I wanted to do was sleep. The room seemed so large and white, but when I see it now while doing hospital visiting it isn't any different than other rooms.

George came to visit toward evening. Afterward he confessed that when I was examined in the Emergency Room the night before he was horrified that I couldn't even lift my legs. My legs and I were no longer communicating and it bothered George far more than it bothered me. By that time, the pain had worn me down to indifference to my increasing paralysis. I had lost the desire to move or to worry about moving.

The next morning, December 26, I was relieved that Christmas Day had come and gone. It was a Christmas that I wanted to put in the past as quickly as possible. A nurse came in with my little wash basin and a fresh washcloth. "Good morning. My name is Stephie. I'll be your nurse today," she smiled. Before I could respond, she produced a little white paper cup and held the water tumbler out for me. "This blue pill is…" I drifted off during the explanation but came awake when I heard "…bladder infection."

So that's why I was nauseous and bloated. That's why I was so thirsty. I remembered the cranberry juice, the wonderful iced cranberry juice.

"Do you think you can go to the bathroom if I help you?"

I nodded, grateful to be given a choice in this nightmare of no control over my life. After I was safely returned to the bed, Stephie told me that after breakfast I would be moving to a smaller room. That room would be needed for something else that I didn't quite understand. I think I was asleep before she finished speaking.

George came and went several times that day but I was barely aware, no doubt making him doubly lonely and afraid. No one had taken him aside to explain my prognosis. We were still going on the breezy assumption given us by Dr. Raymond that I would get it all back, an unlikely seeming prospect at that time. In his panic, George imagined me to be paralyzed forever as I continued to deteriorate.

# 14

## *What I've Learned About GBS*

We have since learned that until deterioration stops prognosis is difficult. My conclusion is that GBS will do what it will do. However, in the past twenty years plasmapherisis, commonly known in the GBS community as washing of the blood, has proven useful in shortening the length and sometimes severity of the ascending stage of paralysis. The procedure actually removes the fluid part of the blood—the plasma. The plasma contains the antibodies that are attacking the protective coating of the nerves (the myelin sheath) thereby causing the pain and paralysis. Each plasmapheresis treatment takes several hours. Some patients say that it tires them out, but people who undergo the series of six to ten treatments seem to have a smoother recovery period. Plasmapherisis should be given, however, sooner rather than later. By the time I was hospitalized the progression of the disease had been ascending for a couple of weeks and myelin sheaths were pretty well destroyed in my legs and right arm.

Another treatment that has recently been successful with GBS is intravenous gamma globulin (IVIg), a high dose solution of proteins called gamma globulins which contain antibodies providing immunity against disease. These antibodies are thought to block the action of the antibodies causing the myelin damage. Again, the decision to use this procedure is up to the doctor. Each case is different and will be treated differently.

I have questioned George closely since my illness and he does not remember anyone giving him many details about Guillain Barre or advising him on treatments. It could be that in his frazzled state, coupled with lack of sleep, facts were not digested. Sometimes printed information is best so it can be studied and absorbed gradually.

Our youngest daughter Alice, meanwhile, was conferring with her Seattle neurologist friend and acquiring a list of questions to ask the doctors in Denver. Talk with the intern or resident, he advised. Ask about diagnosis, recovery, medications, tests, and follow up care such as visiting nurse and physical therapy. Family also needs to be kept informed. They need to know to what to expect and how to care for you at home.

Alice is not shy nor is she reticent about obtaining information. Her conversation with Dr. Axel., one of the residents in the unit, indicated that the diagnosis was consistent with Dr. Raymond's conclusion: atypical inflammatory polyneuropathy—Guillain Barre. My case was considered atypical because the nerve involvement was not symmetrical. My right foot was more affected than the left. Even today, when I'm tired the right foot tends to droop and causes me to trip. I've learned to be very careful and concentrate on picking up my feet. To do that it's best if I don't talk while walking, hold on to the stair rail, and watch for obstacles. I like to joke that my right ankle is a handy weather barometer. Everyone listens when I announce an oncoming storm.

Continuing tests were ruling out diabetes or possible tumor as the cause of the pain. Even at University Hospital the notion of stress still lingered as a likely culprit for the pain until motor and sensory problems developed further. The information that George and I had offered about my teaching and writing workload and my questionable posture at the computer misled everyone, it seems.

Be careful, especially if you are a woman, not to appear mentally or emotionally troubled. Guillain Barre is hard to diagnose and no one case is exactly the same. I have heard of a woman confined in a psychiatric ward before being correctly diagnosed. Fortunately for new patients, pain as a presenting symptom seems to be more in the news the past few years. I have heard many patients speak of pain.

During this time Alice was also gathering valuable facts on GBS and the Guillain Barre Syndrome Foundation International based in Wynnewood, PA. Alice's former college roommate and best friend was working in California as a hospital nurse. Donna had seen enough cases of GBS to be familiar with my symptoms as Alice described them to her. Donna contacted the people at the Foundation and had them send me a brochure. As soon as I was home and beginning to recuperate I sent in a donation and put my name on the mailing list for the GBS Foundation newsletters.

I was too sick at first to understand much of what I was reading, but have since learned a lot from those newsletters. Another earlier name for GBS is Landry's ascending paralysis, so called because the weakness and paralysis begins with the extremities and works up, often to the nerves and muscles that control breathing. At that point a patient must go on a respirator. No wonder, I reflected, that the nurses were so obsessed with measuring my oxygen intake. One night there were oxygen tubes that kept falling out of my nostrils, causing a screeching sound that I found annoying. It seemed like a nurse would immediately rush in and stop the noise. Nurses and aides also took vital signs more often than I thought necessary, especially in the middle of the night. My blood pressure and heart rate were a constant point of fascination for them. Why, I remember wondering, did they have to wheel in that incredibly loud and clumsy looking machine. The rattling and grinding sound soon became part of the daily routine.

I was lucky to be paralyzed only from the waist down. The brochure I read during recovery at home assures that less than five per cent of patients die from this syndrome—called a syndrome because it is a collection of symptoms rather than a specific disease. However, everyone I have met since my time as a patient refers to GBS as a disease. One man I visited in hospital has called it "a fascinating disease." It is that. The defense system of antibodies and white blood cells are triggered into damaging the nerve covering or insulation—the myelin sheath—in the peripheral nerves, those outside the brain and spinal cord. As there is generally no damage to the central nervous system there is more positive outlook for recovery. But getting back to normal does not occur without physical therapy—a lot of physical therapy, as Dr. Raymond had warned.

It turned out that I would be moved after supper that night. I guess hospitals, like everything else, get off schedule at times. My new room would be my home for the next eleven days. There is nothing like a semi private room to enhance one's social life, ready and willing or not. You either get acquainted and get along with your roommate or you make yourself miserable.

As tired and sleepy as I had been for the past twenty-four hours, I was once again fighting insomnia after I was moved into the new room. It is terribly frustrating to be tired beyond all description but be unable to sleep. My roommate had insomnia also and dealt with it by sitting straight up in bed, all lights brightly lit and television on. She was not inclined to chatting. My heart sank. How was I ever going to get through this hideous night?

During commercial breaks on TV, however, this sleepless lady confided that she was going home in the morning. Hooray, I silently cheered. I was too miserable to wonder who would take her place. Toward midnight a nurse came in to check on me. "Can we please turn off some lights?" I had become bold in my desperation for some peace. Some lights went off but the television played on. The next morning I wished my roommate Godspeed as she happily packed her things. I would have four successive roommates during my stay but none like her. Thank you Lord, I prayed, as she was wheeled out of the room.

By Friday, December 27th we were getting down to business. Into my room came a pleasant young man dressed in blue scrubs. "How are you doing today?" Why do they always ask that when you are lying flat on your back unable to move. And just as silly, most of us say *fine*. Once we got past the small talk, it was revealed that this nice young man would be coming by later in the day to give me a spinal tap. *But*, I felt like protesting, *been there-done that*. But of course I remained silent.

Despite having had a spinal tap when I was diagnosed by Dr Raymond at the other hospital, the order had come down for yet another spinal tap. One hospital does not take another hospital's word for anything. Could things have changed that much in those few days. This is where I have observed a lot of needless repetition in procedures and tests, especially when some insurance companies push people from one system to another. Months later, George and I would give thanks for God's good care in protecting us from frustrating bureaucracy. We still had in effect the comprehensive policy IBM was providing its retirees.

My heart sank when I realized that the spinal tap would be administered with no nurse in attendance. What will this nice young man do if something goes wrong? His concern for my comfort was so touching, though, that I found myself reassuring him. The procedure was soon over with not much more discomfort than the first spinal tap. There followed more blood draws and nerve conduction tests before I was pronounced officially GBS. Now I was a bonafide patient in the Neuroscience and Orthopedic Unit of a big city hospital. Physical therapy would begin the next day as the institution began to gear up after the Christmas holiday period.

# 15

## *Morphine is a Dark Lady*

By Friday December 27th I was at my weakest point, physically, mentally, and emotionally. Two therapists visited me that day. Each of them looked young enough to be my daughter, maybe my granddaughter. But looks are deceiving. They were both very competent young women. Occupational therapists, I learned, teach one how to manage everyday tasks while working around—or should I say with—one's disabilities. Among other things I learned how to bring myself to a sitting position, how to swing my legs over the side of the bed and how to hang onto the rails of the bed while summoning help. Privately, I was planning my own strategies.

Then there is the physical therapist, without which no Guillain Barre patient achieves good recovery. I have the utmost respect for physical therapists. They know every muscle, bone and nerve in the human body. They have the ability to prescribe, teach, and monitor precisely the correct exercise or movement to build muscle tone without incurring injury. They also possess healing hands for massaging deep tissue damage, as I would discover in the months to come. Most of all they exhibit patience with hurting and fearful disease victims. They are truly angels on earth. My first physical therapy that day consisted of range of motion exercises. It didn't seem like we were doing much—little more than gentle massage of my feet and hands, but I was exhausted when it was over.

However, by New Year's Day I progressed to toddling down the hall with the walker, the physical therapist at my side, and into a small waiting room that doubled as a miniature PT set up. There we practiced the art of raising one foot to a step, pushing up and off to the next step, gripping the handrail and praying that the therapist would catch me in the likely event I would fall down. I was becoming paranoid about falling. Altogether there were five steps. By the third step Judy was gently urging, "Just one more step, you're doing fine." Toward the end of my hospital stay I became brave enough to progress down the hall by myself. "Look at you!" exclaimed the nurses. I glowed with pride.

George, in the meantime, was communicating with friends and family. The two of us are so different; when I am hurting or upset I retreat within myself and shut off emotionally. He, on the other hand, reaches out to others. Like our youngest daughter Alice, he gathers as much information and advice as he can, then moves to solve the problem. I ignore the problem. My way does not always work, but in these circumstances it was the only thing I could do or was capable of doing. My constant sleepiness was probably only partially due to GBS. The list of drugs ordered for me is staggering when I read it years later.

Usually I think carefully before taking an aspirin. I am susceptible to any substance that induces euphoria. It is a family joke that to give Mom a glass of wine is to lose her for a few hours. So with all the medication I was making a career of sleeping. Visitors came and went, sometimes leaving a note: Dropped by to see you but you were asleep. Didn't want to wake you." *Ha.* When awake I was moaning. No wonder George was alarmed.

What really knocked me out was a late night experience with morphine. That evening I could not get to sleep. I remember there were two night nurses named Linda, one with blond hair and one with brown hair. My bedtime ritual went smoothly under their expert guidance and I always felt that I was in good hands. That night neither one was on duty. That jarred me; I had come to rely on their caring manners. Instead a substitute introduced himself. I was not happy about the idea of having a male nurse oversee my bedtime ritual. *This is not good. What happens if I have to be catherized?* Tension and worry are not good for pain. To top it off, that was the night someone was pushing a rattling cart up and down the hall. I thought with irritation that the hospital must have hired someone specifically to push a cart up and down past my room to keep me awake.

By midnight I couldn't stand it anymore and I pushed the buzzer. When Joe appeared I asked for morphine. Joe was agreeable. As luck would have it, the day nurse and I had just that afternoon decided that I wouldn't need the IV line in my arm anymore. I can get by, I assured her, without any more morphine shots. So here was Murphy's law to prove me wrong.

Joe returned with he shot equipment and began tightening the rubber tubing around my arm. Poking and sticking seemed to go on forever before a likely vein appeared. Finally, the needle went into my arm, the morphine flowed into the vein and I knew only darkness. I waited for it, welcomed it. From a long way off I heard a voice. It seemed to be coming from a room full of white beds laid out in rows. I was lying on one of them. "How is the pain?" the voice asked again. *What pain? Who is he talking to? I should say something.* "There is no pain." From a distance I heard the voice again, "Good." Then came eight hours of oblivion.

Morphine is a dark lady, She blesses with sleep but demands her payment. She has to be treated with respect and care. That morning I awoke with a hangover: nausea, dizziness, blinding headache. The pain from the night before didn't seem so bad compared to the misery of the morning. Then came a terrible thought. *Today I get the tooth patched.* Two nights before in my befuddled state, I had tried to get up in the semi-darkness without reaching for my walker. Naturally, my legs went out from under me and I crashed into a chair. My startled roommate called out, "Are you all right?"

I lied to cover my embarrassment. "I'm OK." Panting with exertion, I struggled to the bathroom, switched on the light and noticed with detachment that one of my front teeth was mostly missing. George almost fainted when he saw me the next day. Now I was scheduled to have the folks at the dental school downstairs put a temporary fix on the tooth. Misery never comes in small batches, I reflected.

Sure enough, an aide soon popped in to announce cheerfully that Transport would arrive shortly to take me downstairs. Transport arrived in the form a large hearty man in blue scrubs. Ignoring my lack of conversation, he helped into a wheelchair and, chatting all the while, whizzed me down the hall and into the elevator. I drooped over the arm of the wheelchair and tried not to think about vomiting. At the clinic two young dental students held me up while my jaw and maybe my whole body were X-rayed. Were visions of lawsuits dancing through someone's head? All I wanted was to lie down and die.

"OK, one directed, "now let's go over here and lie down." *I'm all for that.* "Open your mouth and relax." I closed my eyes and let them have their way with my teeth. George was greatly reassured when he saw me that afternoon—no more gaping hole in the front of my mouth. Months later, my dentist worked valiantly to save what was left of the tooth, and I'm happy to say the tooth is still with me.

That afternoon Kathy was there with my friend Elsie. I struggled to make small talk with them but I could tell from the look on Elsie's face that I must not look so good. Months later Elsie told me, "You could have died." I hadn't thought about that. Fortunately, I had my tooth fixed before she arrived.

Kathy soon knew much of the staff by name. Her experience as a hospital LPN gave her a knowledgeable and easy manner. Combined with her natural outgoing personality, she is an ideal patient advocate. How lucky we were to have her there. She questioned without challenging, observed without interfering. Dr. Jerome Groopman in his book *Second Opinions* says that patients and their families need to be aware that no prognosis or diagnosis is perfect. As health care consumers we need to balance information and intuition for the best possible use of medical resources. An advocate like Kathy is the perfect tool for gathering information and making decisions.

Doctors need not feel challenged by our need to know as much as possible about our conditions. Patients and their health care providers are ideally working as a team. Kathy insisted on looking at my hospital records the day before my discharge. I wouldn't have thought of doing that, nor would George. But if there was something in those records that we had not been aware of, some uncertain prognosis or complication that had not been communicated or understood, we could have found it then. As it was, everything was in order. But it was peace of mind for me while recovering.

# 16

## *Patients' Rights*

I have saved a copy of George's early e-mail to friends and family. He asks for prayers for understanding and knowledge for my caregivers and "patience for the rest of us." He also voices his anger at doctors in general with their lack of problem solving and his frustration on not being able to offer input. It is, he says "frustrating to be told to be quiet and let Ann do all the talking about her symptoms and problems."

George's communiqué does, however, exhibit admiration for the cooperative methods used in a teaching hospital. "This synergetic approach," he says, "is definitely needed for Ann's condition at this time." Teaching hospitals have the advantage of using a team of doctors rather than relying on one person's opinion. This teamwork approach includes seeking information from sources outside one particular hospital. All of this coordinated effort works toward the benefit of the patient.

As in every situation, however, there are disadvantages. If one medical student examines a patient and another comes to the bedside a short while later, the whole routine is repeated: tapping the knees for responses that are not there, commanding a foot to bend when it will not bend, etc. Joseph Heller, in his memoir of being a GBS patient, *No Laughing Matter,* talks about the endless repetitions of muscle tests by trainers and trainees: "It did not occur to me that I could say no. I did not know that often these strangers had nothing to do with my care."

One morning during doctors' rounds, I kept sleeping and no one could wake me. I remember a white-coated figure calling my name over and over. I must have opened one eye. "Are you having trouble waking up today, Mrs. Brandt?" I don't think I answered. If they wanted any conversation that morning they must have been disappointed because when I woke up several hours later, I was alone in the room.

The problems piled up. The food, I told George in a moment of levity, must have been the result of a contest sponsored by a reverse culinary society with the criteria of worst cooking. The city hospital had won hands down. The hospital must have also won Grand Champion for Worst Coffee. Every time a food tray was set before me, I would pick up a fork, uncover the surprise of the day and shudder. Dinners were the worst. I couldn't look at the meat and gravy mixtures set before me.

No one talks much about what GBS does to the digestive system, particularly elimination problems. When bowels and bladder become paralyzed there are big problems. Finally an understanding nurse ordered fruit salads for my evening meals.

People lose weight during GBS from not eating and because their muscles atrophy. I also developed a strange metallic taste which at times made me feel quite nauseated. Others I've talked to have mentioned having had the same problem with that odd taste. However, I didn't lose as much weight as some people I've heard about. Joseph Heller writes about losing more than forty pounds. The muscles atrophy when there are no nerve impulses to control them. In addition, pain and medication cuts appetite to almost nothing. I had to force myself to eat because I didn't want to stay sick.

Another thing I've learned is how variable the onset and symptoms of GBS can be. Sue Baier in her 1985 book *Bed Number Ten* recounts her GBS experience as a patient with one of the worst imaginable cases. Baier's GBS came on suddenly and she was completely paralyzed. With only her eyelids moving she remained helpless from December 1980 until spring of 1981. She was discharged from the hospital a year after onset of what she calls a "wretched disease." Her book is now recommended reading for medical students, not for technical aspects but for understanding the feelings and fears of patients.

Caring and love by and for her family did much to sustain Sue Baier through her ordeal. So it was with me. From the calls and visits by my family and friends to the prayers of our church congregation I felt nurtured and cared for. I don't know how Kathy managed to do everything she did. In the few days she was in town she cleaned the house, cooked and froze meals and took phone calls from relatives who, not having received a Christmas card, corectly assumed something was wrong. She also helped to calm George's nerves when her siblings felt he was "freaking out."

Having Kathy there was peace of mind. I knew that George was not alone and that we had someone with credentials who could talk knowledgeably to the doctors. Kathy is persistent and when she wants to know something she will find out. It is a sad fact but unofficially true that medical personnel will pay more attention to a patient who has family and friends around. The profession is composed of human beings driven by the same psychology as other people. The quiet patient who follows orders, submits to procedures without question, and has no visitors to intervene does not usually demand or receive extra attention.

When no one was in the room and I was half awake, the television was an undemanding companion. Now when I visit patients I understand why the television is almost always on. It's a link with the outside world and requires no response from a weary viewer. It lends a kind of homey touch to an otherwise isolating situation. One can always doze off in the middle of a program and not miss much. In fact, during my recovery at home, I became addicted to a particular daytime "soap" that I still watch faithfully. Most days George watches it with me. Our children regard our Program as a harmless addiction. They look at each other, shrug their shoulders, roll their eyes, and sigh. Such is the way of aging parents, they seem to say.

On New Years Eve Kathy came to spend an evening with me, watching the midnight frenzy in Times Square. I stayed awake until 10:30, then Kathy looked tired and I suggested she go back to the house. It was a pleasant evening. For a while I could forget that my hair was dirty and overgrown and my wardrobe had lately consisted of a choice between pink flowered or blue flowered nighties. The next day would be the first day of 1997 and I wanted to go home. The desire grew stronger with every hour.

A little girl had been murdered in Boulder, the news reporter said on television. I was only beginning to become aware of events outside the hospital. Murder in Boulder? It didn't seem possible What else might be going on that I wasn't aware of? Surely I could cope with all the inconveniences of paralysis at home. It would take another four days to convince the doctors to discharge me to our multi-level house where George would be my sole caregiver.

# 17

## *Preparing for Discharge*

Those days while waiting to be released from the hospital were filled with uncertainty. On the telephone I would tell my family, "When I get home...." Then the sentence would die before it was born. *When I get home when?* Once Guillain Barre has reached its peak, a stage of limbo occurs. This stage is called recovery although it may not seem so to the patient who has been through so much and only wants to be done with the whole miserable business. There is no way to avoid the tedium and discomfort of this stage of GBS.

Even though my case was not severe and I was not intubated (put on a breathing machine) at any time, recovery was painful and slow. In weeks to come at home as the nerves in my feet and legs began coming back to life, the feeling of pins and needles intensified to the point where I could not bear the weight of a blanket, especially at the end of the day. This posed a dilemma as I could not seem to get warm enough for comfort.

As discharge day drew near the process dragged out. A new room-mate was installed in the bed near the window. This would be the fourth roommate, not counting the night owl of the first night. This one was totally bedridden so there was no competition for the bath-room which was just as well because the process used to determine if I had any heavy metals in my body was cumbersome and took up a lot of space in the bathroom. Every bit of liquid going into my body and coming out had to be measured and examined. Some day I intend to find out why, but I'm too busy living my life at this moment.

Meanwhile, my anxiety about what was going on at home mounted. This state of uncertainty was heightened when Kathy dropped a casual sentence into the tedium of an afternoon. "You should see the dining room soffit."

*Oh no. Now what is he doing?* After more than four decades of marriage, I had come to expect the unexpected when George began to unleash his creative side. We had remodeled the whole first floor of the house the year before and the spacious shelf nine feet above the dining room had been an object of my decorating dreams, made and discarded over the months. Evidently the soffit was no longer bare and virgin, awaiting the fine hand of the mistress of the house. "What about the soffit?"

"Oh, dad was up there arranging and rearranging. It's a flower garden now."

I gulped. There was nothing I could do. I would have to wait and see. My distress worsened when Kathy described the living room as a duster's nightmare. *What is that man doing with the house?* Clutter frays my nerves. George and I had always had a traditional division of chores at home. He has kept things working and I have kept things running. We don't usually intrude in each other's domains. It sounded like all control was lost. I almost dreaded going home to face the unknown.

Meanwhile things at home were getting busy. Kathy had to reassure George that I wouldn't be paralyzed forever the day he went into a panic and announced he would have to sell the house and get a place with no stairs. (Now I use our three flights of stairs as a kind of physical therapy on days it's too cold or wet to go out walking.) Kathy, Pastor Brad, and George worked the day before my homecoming to rearrange furniture for my complete comfort in our garden level master bedroom. The room would be my prison and my retreat for the next several months, although I did find a way to maneuver up and down on a limited basis. Kathy was especially careful to lay in a supply of food for snacks in case I got hungry. It seemed that my lack of appetite had folks worried. However, GBS does dull the zest for food and many patients lose more than the ten or so pounds I dropped.

Getting me from point A to point B any amount of distance was going to be a problem in the near future. My dear friend Mary had a wheelchair she had used for her elderly aunt. It was old and very basic, not like some of the electronic marvels I had seen buzzing up and down the corridors of Front Range College. I remember that one of my students had a wheelchair that tipped back and forth, swiveled, and ran on her choice of several speeds. Very nice and very pricey. Mine would be more basic, but we could use it for as long as we needed. Mary and Ray delivered it to the house before I came home.

When the work crew finished with my homecoming preparations, the wheelchair sat folded up in the middle of the living room, propped up beside Lucky's large dog crate, brought upstairs from its usual spot in our bedroom. Lucky would be without a definite place to spend the night, wandering instead from George's side in the upstairs guestroom to my quarters two flights down. She was a very confused dog for a while.

The strange ambiance of the living room was further enhanced by the few Christmas decorations I had set in place before I got sick, and by the rows of figurines—ceramic teddy bears, angels, quasi Hummels, real Hummels—prize finds from George's many stress relieving shopping trips. It was worse than I could have imagined. A week later, through connections with my friend Shirley, we obtained the services of a thorough cleaning woman. She came in one day and swept through the house like a cleansing breeze. George couldn't find anything for several days afterward, but I was thrilled.

The morning of discharge day finally arrived. The day nurse came into the room to give me written instructions and a list of my medications. When I view the list now, I'm not surprised that I spent so much time in recovery asleep. The day before discharge, Rita had taught me how to insert my own catheter if needed. I prayed not to need it. There was some last minute discussion about which doctor to see for follow up visits. So many doctors had seen me in the hospital, it seemed no one doctor was in charge of my case. I suspect that was a problem stemming from being admitted through the emergency room with no official physician—no "attending doctor." We hadn't learned the lingo or the ways of the system, even then.

As I had seen Dr. Widrow that first day and he had been on rounds several times during the past few days, Rita and I decided to put his name on the discharge sheet. He and his staff would be a bit surprised when George made an appointment and brought me to his office a week later. It seems that George and I had not only not followed the system but we had thrown it out altogether. Will you be OK at home, Rita wanted to know.

"I'm a strong minded woman," I assured her. I would have time to remember those words in the long and lonely weeks to come.

# 18

## *Homecoming-The Agony and the Ecstasy*

Saturday January 4 was a big day for me: becoming a person again, wearing clothes instead of flowered, tie-back nighties. It seemed strange to be wearing clothes again like a normal person even though all my jewelry was at home. I would reclaim that part of myself too. *I'll be an independent woman.* Once outside the hospital on the way to the car I felt like calling out to passersby from my wheelchair, "Hello world!"

As the car slowed to a stop in the driveway the front door burst open and Kathy hurried out to meet us. "Hi Mom!" It was like I had never been gone except that I was stuck in the car and needed help getting out. It took some time to get me out of the front seat. George and Kathy each took one of my legs, heavy cumbersome things that flopped around like newly caught fish. Finally we got my feet on the ground and my husband and my eldest daughter half carried me into the house. The excitement and the physical activity had worn me out, but I pulled together all of my remaining strength to help them get me down the stairs to the master bedroom that would become my haven and my prison in the following weeks.

I sank down on the foot of the bed, too tired to think of removing my coat. I don't even remember Kathy leaving; she had a plane to catch and a family waiting for her in Tucson. The next day I would call Scott and thank him for lending us his wife. She was a lifesaver.

I arrived home at 11:00am. When I woke up it was 3:00pm. George grinned as he helped me off with my coat. "You fell asleep. The physical therapist and the visiting nurse will be here soon." Sure enough. Almost on cue Lucky began barking. Two cars were out in front of the house, one with the physical therapist and one with the visiting nurse.

When George answered the doorbell and led them down the stairs, my spirits sank when I saw that the RN was a male nurse. I remembered Joe from the night of the midnight morphine. But this person soon proved to be very knowledgeable. Morphine, he told George, can be quite effective if used wisely. He went on to explain the half-life of the drug and how it can be administered in increments to stay within the safe level, relieve pain, and keep pain under control. We must not expect to be completely pain free, but to keep the pain from building to a crescendo we need a level amount in our bloodstream. I was still too foggy to absorb much of what was said, but that information proved quite valuable to George as my caregiver.

The therapist did a quick evaluation of my physical abilities and limitations, giving hints on how to get out of bed, sit upright in a chair, walk with my walker. When we toured the bathroom I asked what was utmost in my mind at that moment. "Is there any way I can have a bath?" A shower was out of the question. The step into it was too risky and I could imagine crashing into the glass sides. The bath tub was another puzzle. *I might be able to get into it, maybe.* But getting out, Linda reminded me would be a big problem. I had to agree; the idea of a rescue team coming into the bathroom to extract me from the tub didn't sound appealing. I guess sponge baths would have to do for a while longer, I thought, resigned. Linda promised to come back in two days to begin my exercises. The nurse wished us good luck. Our insurance would pay for one visit from him. We were alone to begin the adventure of GBS recovery.

A short time later, Norm and Lois from our church brought over enough food for several meals, so I knew George would have enough to eat. Food was still repellent to me. After supper George studied the list of medications and the times I was to get them. How much sleep would he get that night? Not much, it turned out.

Discharge instructions called for my last medications of the day to be given at 10:00pm and the first ones at 6:00am with Tylox/oxycodeine every four to six hours as needed for pain. It sounded all right on paper. George tucked me into bed, left a night light on and made sure my walker was handy. He had bought me a floppy cloth doll with blond pigtails toward the end of my hospital stay. All the nurses admired her as she grinned from her perch above my bed. I named her Griswelda. So I hugged Griswelda tight and closed my eyes.

Pain again, growing like an evil monster. I couldn't help moaning. It was dark even with the nightlight. George appeared time and time again. He gave me the Tylox. Throughout the night we cheated on the time until it was less than three hours between doses. Each time I moaned George was at my side in his pajamas. "Where are you sleeping?" I knew that he couldn't possibly hear me from the bedroom two floors up.

"Never mind," he said.

Why is that pain visits at night? I slept most of Sunday. That evening our good friends Don and Sandy and Joann and George arrived with a meal——again enough for several meals. George was going to have start putting some of this food in the freezer. I loved the feeling of being fed and nurtured. They brought a plant, too, and I instructed George to put it with the Christmas arrangement that Shirley and Tom had sent over when I was in the hospital. I normally don't like being fussed over, but now the feeling of being cared for and loved almost made up for the nightmare of the past weeks.

Evening deepened and so did pain. Remembering what the nurse had said about issuing a half dose of morphine and staying comfortable, I got an idea. Of course I should have had that idea 24 hours before but neither George nor I had been thinking clearly. "Morphine," I said. George looked dubious. I persisted. "We don't want to have a repeat of last night do we?" He was convinced.

It seemed no doctor at University Hospital wanted to be in charge of ordering morphine for an outpatient. George had to go down there in person to pick up the prescription and get it filled at an all night pharmacy—one that carried morphine. "You can't stay here alone." True, I was almost totally helpless and afraid to be alone. Then I thought of Terri, my friend who had taken such good care of me on Christmas Eve.

Terri used to always take the night shift at Boulder Community Hospital when all of our children were young, so she was home during the day. I'll never forget the time that Shirley next door and I were both at work and all of our boys decided to concoct something in Shirley's kitchen. Something happened with knives that resulted in a lot of blood and frightened boys. Terri was there with first aid and ready to soothe distraught mothers when we found out about the adventure. Everyone should plan to raise children in a neighborhood where a nurse lives nearby.

Terri arrived and we settled in for an evening of waiting and praying while George was out on slippery streets in a blinding snowstorm with only one headlight operating on the car. It's a good thing we didn't know all the details of what he was going through. Eleven o'clock came and went. Terri and I covered many topics of conversation. In between talking she rubbed my back. "It feels like your nerves are jumping up and curling around my finger," she said. But Terri's acupressure brought a measure of relief. Looking back, that comment makes a lot of sense; if nerves are being attacked naturally pain will be involved. Pain in GBS is a topic that needs a lot more attention.

Midnight came and we began to worry. To keep our spirits up we started telling jokes, corny at first then slightly off color jokes, laughing heartily to keep from crying. Just as we were reacting to another story with forced laughter, we heard the front door upstairs. "Hello! Are you girls awake?" At that moment I loved George more than any time since I could remember. "You can't believe what they had me doing."

It turned out that he had to go from hospital to drugstore and back several times because of the complications in obtaining a controlled substance at an odd hour. I remember the days when we gave babies paregoric for stomachache. We all slept much better in those days. Paregoric is no longer an over the counter drug.

So we settled into a routine of sorts. The liquid morphine (Roxane) would be administered with an eyedropper. It tastes unbelievably bitter. It's a good idea to keep a supply of hard candy nearby. After a dose of Roxane a lemon drop is a welcome relief. Following what the RN had said, I had half the Roxane about seven in the evening. Then at about ten or eleven just before bed, I would have the other half dose. That allowed a relatively fair night's sleep, for both of us. George kept track of the rest of the medications, giving them out at proper daytime intervals.

Another problem stalked us. It wasn't me; it was George. He was still plagued with bronchitis even though he had given up smoking in November. Worse yet, he had a red rash on both thighs, painful and itchy. Shingles, said the doctor. From stress. It was a light case but fatigue had already begun to drag at George's energy. Care givers worry, do without sleep, and are on call for any emergency. They are responsible for the comfort, safety and happiness of the patients. And George has always taken responsibility seriously. Now that I was home and he had mastered the art of laundry, shopping and cooking, life was under some semblance of control. But the ordeal of the past weeks had taken its toll.

On Tuesday, George felt comfortable enough to leave me alone for the morning while he kept his doctor appointment. I'll be OK, I assured him. I can always call Terri. But I was so cold. George had brought a portable electric heater from his workshop down to the bedroom and I turned it up to maximum level. Temperature in the hospital hadn't been a problem because hospitals seem to keep their rooms extra hot in the winter. (Summers are another matter; rooms are almost at a freezing level.) I've heard of abnormal sensations in GBS patients and I guess body temperature going out of control one way or the other can be included in the category of abnormal sensations.

According to information we have found on the Internet, when the immune system begins to destroy the myelin sheath surrounding the nerve cell axons the nerves cannot transmit signals efficiently. This is the underlying cause of tingling, numbness and paralysis. Because nerve signals to and from the arms and legs must travel the longest distances they are most vulnerable to interruption. That is why weakness and tingling generally first appear in the hands and feet.

On the other hand, nerve signals are sometimes mixed up and the brain may receive inappropriate signals that result in a feeling of things crawling on the skin, even painful sensations. No two cases of GBS are alike, making it difficult to diagnose the disease in its early stages. I've talked to many GBS patients who have experienced pain to one degree or another both during the acute phase and during recovery. The medical community has only recently beginning to talk of pain as a symptom of Guillain Barre. I visited a patient whose midsection kept remembering the feeling of the belt used to fasten her to the tilt table during one of her treatments. Her nerves, the therapist had joked, were confused and trying to figure out what to do with the sensation. I remember the patient and I chuckling over that remark.

Meanwhile I was apprehensive about moving around the room for fear of falling and nobody to help me up. I probably would have mustered enough strength and courage to pull myself up, though. My little mantra had become *I WILL do this.* Is this why we need to worry when a patient is too acquiescent? I have often wondered about this issue. As the room seemed to grow colder, I turned up the setting on the portable heater that George had brought down for me. As it grew later, I became more anxious for his return. Tomorrow my real adventures would begin.

# 19

## *Wheelchair Adventures*

It was time to find out what it's like to be confined to a wheelchair. A sense of humor is a vital ingredient for this adventure.

After lunch and my nap, George announced that he had found a great deal on reclining chairs on the way home from the doctor yesterday. How many reclining chairs I had the foresight to ask, remembering the case of pineapple in the pantry from one of his recent excursions. "Six," he replied, then launching into a description and the merits of each one.

Six recliners! It seemed a bit much. But, George explained in a reasonable tone, two for each floor. Just like a walker on each floor—from one of his other previous shopping trips. My husband never does things half way. Would I come and look at them, he inquired. I was dressed, sort of. Even early in my convalescence I tried to put on casual clothing for at least part of the day. I had had enough of continuous nightgowns in the hospital. And I certainly was not going to receive visitors in my nightie. Visitors are an important part of recovery for GBS patients, at least this patient.

So, we set forth, me in my velour lounging outfit and my big fuzzy slippers. Shoes at this stage were out of the question as my feet were swollen and felt like lumps of clay held together at the ankles with tight rubber bands. My fingers didn't work enough to manage putting on my own socks as yet either. The weather was cold and snow threatened but we got me into the car, with a heavy jacket over my improvised daytime outfit. The old borrowed wheelchair was stowed away in the trunk of the car and we were off.

It is a bit of a project to unpack a wheelchair, help the patient out of the car, hold everything steady for the transfer in the wheelchair and proceed into the store. I tried to ignore the stares I imagined were coming my way. We trundled over the icy parking lot and into the store. *This thing sure rattles.* I was tired already. After much discussion about this or that feature on several chairs, I was becoming thirsty. Where, I asked, might I find a water fountain. Right over by that wall, the salesman informed me. So I rattled off in the wheelchair to the other end of the store. The average drinking fountain is not designed for a person in a wheelchair. Sending up a quick prayer for a shot of strength, I half lifted myself a foot or so off the seat of the chair and caught enough of the water to quench my thirst. Trying to maintain my dignity, I wiped the water spray off my face. *How annoying.*

By the time our business concluded in the furniture store, it was late, dark, and cold. In a burst of enthusiasm over my first outing we decided to stop at a restaurant for a bite to eat. There are times when a woman does not fret about her appearance. This was one of those times. We knew the drill: George run around the car to remove the wheelchair from the trunk, unfold it, bring it to my side of the car, lock the brakes—very important—and remove crippled lady from passenger seat. Unlock brakes, lock car, and trundle into the restaurant. No sooner did we get inside than the right wheel quit on the job. It was an old wheelchair and the tires were ready to fall off. Where else but in a public place with ten or twelve people trying to walk past. No point thinking about dignity.

Somehow we made it to a table. I began to think about how my fuzzy slippers must look and the fact that wheelchairs stick out into the aisles of busy restaurants. The server didn't seem to mind having to walk around me, though. And the curious stares from other patrons turned to friendly smiles. I began to relax. Soon it was time to visit the restroom. This is where I found out how a handicapped person uses a non-handicap stall. After looking over the situation I finally decided on raising myself up, clinging to the doorframe, swaying into the stall, and leaving the wheelchair outside. Of course this blocked access to the wash basins for two other ladies but everyone was accommodating and pleasant.

My anxious husband was hovering outside the ladies room when I emerged in my lopsided wheelchair. Sometimes there is nothing to do but laugh. Norman Cousins got himself over a fatal disease that way after all. So laughing all the way we got in the car and drove home through what was by now a blinding snow storm. Oh and did I mention that we had Lucky the dog in the car with us all this time, panting, slobbering and steaming up the windows.

The next day George the problem solver set out to find a replacement wheel for Old Bessie, the name I had given the wheelchair. After searching through the Yellow Pages and calling various establishments he finally located a place in Denver that sells replacement parts for medical devices. Old Bessie had broken down while in our possession and it is not our policy to borrow something and return it broken. So for the rest of my wheelchair time we had a brand new right wheel.

On Saturday the new recliners were delivered just after the lumpy old sofas were taken away to be given to charity. As dubious as I had felt initially it was nice to have two comfortable upholstered chairs in the master bedroom. I was still confined down there and needed to sit in something besides the hard wooden chair where Linda had given me sitting and standing lessons several days before.

So another routine developed. George brought supper for both of us downstairs, set it up on folding trays, and together we would spend a pleasant evening, eating, chatting, and watching television. A warm feeling enveloped me, and I felt safe and loved. The soft lamplight shone on all of our familiar things. Pictures of our grandchildren filled one section of the wall by our bed. It was so good to be home where I belonged. I felt free to heal. George and I had been together for so many years that constant conversation was not necessary; just his presence was comforting.

As much as I loved having company, being with people for long periods of time was exhausting. I remember going to church for the first time; being in a roomful of people after days of comparative solitude was almost overwhelming. I have never liked noise, and the sounds of many people talking at once was like gunfire to my nerves. I was more than ready to clump with my walker to the car. George had parked in the space marked with the universal sign of a wheelchair. It felt strange to park in a spot that I had always regarded as reserved for old people (I am not young) or crippled people (I couldn't walk unaided). Suddenly I had joined a group of people that always seemed to move in a different world than me. It was a humbling thought.

Getting a handicap placard was easy. George picked up a form at our local automobile licensing office and the doctor filled it out and signed it. The placard didn't cost anything extra and it has been one of the biggest blessings ever since when we need to go where the parking spaces will be far from our ultimate destination. In the state of Colorado the placard goes where the patient goes so I can take my placard along when we visit our children or go out with non-handicapped friends. I only limp when I'm extra tired, but I'm self conscious about not limping when I walk away from my handicapped parking place. There exists a strange combination here of guilt over using a handicap spot and a sense of relief that I have that option. I often wonder how many other people with invisible or barely perceptible handicaps use those special parking spaces and receive grudging stares from the able bodied. Invisible handicaps can be hard for able bodied people to understand.

Going out in public, however, was worth the challenge to me. One episode that George and I remember with fondness is the night we dared to venture to a dinner theater. During my hospital stay a letter had arrived from the City of Broomfield. Congratulations, it said, you are chosen to serve on the library board of trustees and are invited to the mayor's annual dinner at Heritage Square in Golden.

I don't like to miss things. So off we went on the appointed evening. To be absolutely rested I had taken two naps that day. Choosing what to wear on my feet was challenging. Sore and swollen feet do not lend themselves to glamorous shoes. By that time I had started on outpatient physical therapy at Mapleton Rehabilitation Center in Boulder, Colorado. Jill, my therapist there had given me a plastic foot brace to insert in my right shoe, not very fashionable looking but it helped to keep my weak ankle from buckling. My foot had a tendency to flop forward and the brace helped to keep it at an angle that saved me from tripping. Without the brace, I would be stubbing my toe many times in the following months. So I settled for a pair of old sneakers with the laces untied. *Maybe no one will look at my feet.*

But there was an upside. A year before Kathy had given me a chic red jumpsuit. However, it had looked better on the hanger than it did on my body. Now I zipped up the front and it fit loosely. With satisfaction I cinched the wide belt into place and almost toppled over admiring myself in the mirror. Out of adversity does come some advantage I reflected.

Then it was time for the wheelchair routine again. We arrived at Heritage Square early and secured a choice parking place not far from the bottom of the hill we would have to climb to get to get to the Playhouse—or should I say George would have to climb. I sat in the wheelchair providing encouragement and frequent offers to get out and walk. My words fell on deaf ears. He just kept puffing and pushing. Out of the corner of my eye I noticed an icy patch and wondered briefly how it would be going down again.

Some buildings are not yet equipped for wheelchairs and disabled people. Not everything has been revamped according to regulation. To get to the dining room we had to use the stairs. It was that or forgo dinner. As skimpy as my appetite had been, by the end of February I was starting to eat respectable amounts. So we stowed the wheelchair in the coatroom and unfolded the walker brought along for this possibility. Clump, step, clump, step. People either streamed past me or patiently waited in back of me. The latter was making me nervous.

All went well. People I hadn't seen in months exclaimed over my condition and asked the inevitable question—what happened to you. Explaining Guillain Barre over and over to people who have never heard of it becomes tiring. Many people have never heard the word and I was becoming quite practiced with the French accent on the last syllables. The Heritage Playhouse melodrama as usual was entertaining, and it was good to be out with people. I had been told that an enjoyable social life stimulates recovery and wards off depression that can overcome patients in isolation. But in spite of my extra rest during the day, by evening's end I was exhausted and more than ready to go home.

I clumped down the stairs and George retrieved the wheelchair from where he had checked it in the coatroom. I settled in with the walker in my lap, George took control at the handlebars and we were off. Going down a steep hill goes much more swiftly than going up and no encouraging words were needed. Then we came to that icy patch I had noticed earlier.

The pace picked up considerably. Can George control the situation, I wondered in a slight panic. He seemed to be breathing harder. Did I hear the wheels whining on the ice? *Gosh, we're doing some trick wheelchair driving here.* Wind whipping my hair, we whizzed past folks walking leisurely to their cars. George barely keeping up with the wheelchair, we arrived at our car in short order. By that time we were both laughing so hard, that we had gathered a small audience. I still wonder how much George's feet touched the ground on that trip down the hill. The next day as I related that incident to each of our children on four separate telephone calls, I laughed so hard they could barely understand my words. I was disappointed when they didn't share my merriment… "You could have been killed," was the dour comment of one of them. The poor dears had been under so much stress they had lost their sense of humor, I thought.

Wheelchairs can be serious business also. One instance in a department store gave me empathy for people who are stuck in wheelchairs for life. I had maneuvered around the women's clothing section searching for some loose slacks to wear while recuperating. With my selection draped across my lap, I approached the cashier. Ahem, I had to say a couple of times before she looked down. Then I had to stretch up to hand her my charge card. I felt like a child.

Knowing that my wheelchair was a temporary companion I had a bit of fun with the situation. We soon ventured out to the supermarket. George insisted that I use one of those motorized chairs provided by many establishments. Driving one of those things takes practice. On my first try I took out an end display of canned goods. *How embarrassing*. People can be forgiving, however. A clerk appeared almost at once. Brushing aside my offers to pick everything up (empty words because how would I do it) he patiently began restoring the display.

Early in my reentry to shopping I learned that pushing a shopping cart was easier than using my walker. I had insisted on having a walker without wheels—the kind that goes clump, clump. The first walker I had in the hospital had wheels which made it hard for me to control my speed. The domino effect there was the falling down of me. So by process of elimination in reviewing my successes and failures in locomotion, I stayed with either shopping carts or store wheelchairs.

People stare. There is no denying it. Eventually I had enough strength to clump from the handicap parking space to the store. Once inside, however, I knew that I could not navigate any further so George would settle me into the store wheelchair. We knew which stores had them available and which stores had only the motorized versions that we would have to stand in line to get the key for. I really didn't trust myself to be a safe driver in those things any way after the toppled display incident. More than once I noticed people staring as I stood up and walked away from the wheelchair. Charlatan, I could imagine them thinking. Faker. Therein lay some of my guilt. Maybe that's why I concentrated so on having fun and laughing about wheelchairs.

My next wheelchair adventure involved our dog. I had been thinking what a great therapy dog Lucky would be after all her practice in comforting the sick, namely me. What would she do, I wondered, if she had to pull me in the wheelchair. For anyone who might be wondering what their dog would do in similar circumstances, I advise not trying it. Fortunately my experiment was done close to the curb of a deserted parking lot so the crash wasn't too abrupt. Lucky thought the wheelchair was chasing her and she acted accordingly. I don't believe that dogs are cut out to pull wheelchairs.

A memorable evening was the night we went to the theatre. We subscribe to season tickets at the Arvada Theatre less than ten miles from our house and had been attending five times a year with Mary and Ray. I didn't want to miss the performance nor did I want to miss the chance to spend time with friends even though I was only four weeks out of the hospital. When I thought of the staircase that comes into view as soon as one enters the front door, I called ahead to find out the alternate plan for getting to the second floor auditorium. Just the thought of ascending the fifty-two stairs wore me out. Our handicap placard assured that we could park right in front of the building, but George would have to do the wheelchair scene again.

Ray and Mary arrived at our house early to allow extra time for the wheelchair, walker routine. I had taken two naps that afternoon but in the excitement I would have tripped over our front doorstep if not for Ray holding one arm and George holding the other arm. All went well: get the patient out of the car and into the chair, roll around to the entrance on the side of the building, take the elevator up. Then came the tricky part. The usher for our section was a white haired lady who looked like she might be more frail than I was. Much to my chagrin, she took my arm and slowly walked down to our row while I clutched the railing on the wall. My wheelchair was neatly stowed in the back of the auditorium.

When the play was over, before I could wonder where it was, there came my wheelchair with another usher ready to help me into it.

Another usher took my arm to help the process while George and Ray hovered anxiously, ready to lend a hand. After I was seated, the house manager appeared to make sure all went well. I felt like a queen. The whole affair was quite satisfactory and great therapy.

# 20

## *Such Fatigue!*

When I reached the point where I could concentrate enough to read and comprehend information I began to study the newsletter sent by the Guillain Barre Syndrome Foundation International. As a layperson I didn't know where to look for answers to all my questions and the newsletter was a good place to start. The Winter 1996 issue of *The Communicator* contained highlights of the fourth international symposium held in Miami, Florida the previous October. Hmm, I thought, what a long distance to travel for a symposium. I think differently about such things now.

The center pages of the newsletter showed pictures of some of the symposium attendees. Everyone seemed to be having a good time, but I noticed that a few people were in wheelchairs and some were using canes. That puzzled me because didn't patients "get it all back" as I had been told. I decided not to dwell on it and turned to the back cover and the display of items for further reading. That's where I found the title for a couple of books, including *Bed Number Ten*. Also on that page I saw a listing for an online support group for CIDP. Not knowing what those letters symbolized, I skipped to the last item on the list—Bereavement group. This was slightly unnerving. I decided not to think about it.

Since that time I have learned that CIDP is an acronym for Chronic Inflammatory, Demylinating Polyneuropathy. A small percentage of patients suffer with periodic recurrence of symptoms much like arthritis. It is the most discouraging of all conditions in this disease family, but new methods of control are being used with greater and greater success. I have found that the Foundation newsletter contains the most informative literature for the average layperson. At the beginning of my recovery, I found it hard to concentrate, therefore, not understanding much of what I read, but now I read and save all issues and refer back to them periodically.

Research continues on this neurological condition, but the disease is rare and so does not attract the research dollars that other more commonly known afflictions currently pull in. Approximately 7,000 cases are diagnosed in the United States each year with much higher rates in China, Mexico and others. Each case is different in its symptoms, length of onset, and recovery period. As many general care physicians don't see more than one or two cases in their entire practice, it remains difficult to recognize unless the patient is seen by a neurologist. It has been said that medical schools devote an average of one hour of lecture time to Guillain Barre.

In my quest to learn more about GBS I found much of what I was seeking on the Internet. The Foundation maintains a recently updated web site that includes a discussion board where people can trade information and experiences. The web site furnished by the GBS Foundation also includes information on contacting your local support group. The brochure that came in the mail with my first newsletter states that the Foundation exists to "support, educate, and research." Most impressive is that most of the people involved with the Foundation are volunteers. The honorary board includes Joseph Heller (now deceased), author of *Catch 22,* and Andy Griffith. The organization was started in 1980 by Estelle and Robert Bensen as Robert was recovering from GBS. Estelle reflects that during that time, she had no one to turn to for information. At that time she decided that no one should have to go through GBS alone. Dr. Joel Steinberg was also recovering from GBS at that time and together with the Bensens they began organizing the Foundation. An impressive list of neurologists and researchers now comprises the medical board, most of whom speak at the biannual symposia.

Since attending my first symposium in November 2,000 I have gained knowledge and empathy for patients who have been stricken far more severely than I was. I have visited with people using canes and wheelchairs. I have talked with men and women who are left with residual effects both visible and invisible. The airy reassurance that we will get it all back seems a mockery in the face of this evidence to the contrary. While patients need to cling to hope and to have reassurance and support from their medical teams, they also have a right to honesty.

There is indeed a fine line between squashing patients' hopes for recovery and giving patients false hope for a magic cure. That dilemma exists with every serious disease. But each doctor should find out how much information the patient and the caregiver want. Conversely, patients and their families need to realize that no matter how technically skillful and how compassionate doctors are, physicians aren't mind readers. Open and honest two way communication is absolutely essential.

The front cover of that first newsletter I saw featured a letter from Foundation president Estelle Bensen. She speaks of the twenty-two symposium workshops on various aspects of GBS given by professionals in the medical field: "…one of the presenters, a prominent neurologist…after having had the opportunity to speak with so many GBS patients, his approach to treating future patients is going to change. The needs, fears, and concerns surfaced and could not be ignored."

As with any life altering disease, patients need to know that they are not alone, that others have suffered as they have and sometimes more. Some people want to know as much medical detail as they can find. Others simply want to compare notes with others. Most need to know how to live with their disabilities, large and small. Of all GBS survivors I have spoken with, the overwhelming effect of having had GBS is fatigue or reduced stamina.

Fatigue plagued me from the start. It ran a close second to pain. Fatigue is with me still. GBS survivors learn how to pace themselves.

This necessity gives us a new sense of priorities and we learn to ration our efforts to what is most important to us. I used to dash headlong through each day, never thinking about rationing energy. Now I like to think of this new way of living as life enhancement.

However, I—like others—sometimes chafe at the restrictions imposed by having had GBS. It is so easy to tell others to pace themselves, but how impatient I become when I can have one day of what I consider normal activity then pay for it with overwhelming fatigue. Sometimes I feel like all of my energy is flowing out from the soles of my feet. There were times even in my early recovery phase when I felt setbacks in regaining my strength. I know now that recovery can be a recursive process; something gained one day is not around the next day. To patients eager to resume normal living this can be extremely frustrating. So I chugged on, holding myself back one day, sinking with exhaustion another day.

# 21

## *Physical Therapy and Recovery*

As winter deepened time seemed to stand still. The bedroom windows looked out to a tree in the neighbor's yard, home to a family of squirrels. For the first time in my life I found myself studying the activities of squirrels. I had thought only of squirrels as pesky little rodents with big tails, best left alone and ignored. But that winter I observed with interest their various habits. I took note of the way they would curl their tails over their backs to protect themselves from the wind and how they would balance themselves on the telephone wires, sometimes hanging upside down like circus aerial performers. Squirrels are playful, I found. Or maybe they were just running around to keep from freezing to death in one spot.

When the squirrels weren't using the tree for their aerobics the birds moved in and I found myself becoming fascinated with the variety of winter birds in our area. In all my years I had never imagined becoming a bird watcher but there I was, taking an interest in the most miniscule things of nature. I stared with fascination at the tree branches, bare and dark against the winter landscape. There is a time for every season, I thought, and a period of standing still. As I looked at the tree I thought how things in nature know to rest. Did I know how to rest? God had surely gotten my attention and caused me to pause when I wouldn't slow down on my own.

By the end of April I was taking half the amount of morphine dosage and soon ceased to need the evening dose altogether. Pain had faded to discomfort which could be controlled with a heating pad on my back. Instead of feeling tied down to one spot, I would heat up the pad, disconnect it, and tie it around my middle to cover the most sensitive place on my back. There are other products on the market which would work as well or better, but for me at that time it was sufficient.

Physical therapy continued as an outpatient at the Mapleton Rehabilitation Center in Boulder. How I loved easing my body into a pool filled with 90 degree water. When the bottoms of your feet are tender it pays to wear pool shoes. Sporting goods stores sell them or you can wear soft-soled clean slippers. Thong shoes haven't worked for me since I began this GBS adventure because my feet can't keep them on.

Water gives extra buoyancy and once I had crept down the gentle ramp, holding onto the handrail, I would bounce-walk over to the ledge and sit down in front of the water jets for an automatic back massage. I was really taken with the idea of back massage in those recovery days.

Post Guillain Barre physical therapy avoids the no pain-no gain idea and approaches the patient with gentle stretching and stimulation of nerves. Our insurance had allowed a modest sum for renting a small portable nerve stimulator to use on my feet and legs but we bought the unit outright on the theory that it would be good to have around for a long period. I still bring it out from time to time.

My first out patient physical therapy appointment on February 25 began with an evaluation, which is common, so the therapist can plan the best program. My therapist was outstanding: cheerful, sympathetic, and capable all rolled into one. Best of all she was bossy, just the ticket for someone as recalcitrant and stubborn as I. "Just sit on the ledge and start warming up," she directed on my first day in the pool." I obeyed without hesitation.

How pampered I felt when the session was over and I crept up the ramp, hanging onto the rail, to be greeted by a smiling attendant with a large white towel that had been preheated. The whole experience felt more like being in a spa than a rehabilitation facility. But as I looked around and saw therapists working with individual patients I knew how lucky I was. Unlike some of the other patients, I could move my torso and arms, my mind and sense of humor were functioning and my legs were slowly coming back.

After six weeks Jill and the insurance company felt I had progressed enough to manage physical therapy on my own. She gave me homework. I had some basic stretching and toning exercises to practice at home and in the pool during the public swim hours. That wonderful warm water continued its soothing spell. As I went through the sessions I couldn't help thinking what an important role physical therapists play in recovery from any serious illness. They need to focus on the mechanics of what they're doing as well as continually gauge the patient's mental and physical state in order to pace the sessions appropriately. Physical therapists are special people—compassionate and capable.

When my shoulder froze up a couple of years after recovery it was found that I had suffered a small fracture in falling down the stairs that awful night before diagnosis. I could have surgery or physical therapy. Without further discussion I chose therapy. Jill once again developed a regimen of exercises for me. Also, she threw herself into breaking down the calcium buildup between my joints. "This is my fifth soft tissue damage case today," she said, puffing slightly between firm pushes on my shoulder area."

On the premise that a therapist needs moral support while working on one such as me, I would try to find the humorous side of things. "So this job is in place of going to the gym?" I asked as she paused for breath.

"Something like that."

I never stopped looking for the humorous aspects of each session. During one of my in-home appointments I couldn't stop laughing long enough to stay focused on the assignment of the day. The task seemed impossible. Linda had brought in a large sturdy ball two feet in diameter. I had watched her wrestle it from her car and carry it across the street and up to my door. She put it down on the living room floor and I must have looked surprised. There it sat, looming at me. "Today we're going to try something different," she announced.

I looked at the ball with distrust. *This is different all right.* Lucky was already circling the ball, sniffing. George was in the kitchen baking cookies so we might all celebrate the end of the session in good style. "Lie down on the ball, face down," she directed.

*You've got to be kidding.* But I was game. Never let it be said I wouldn't at least try. I placed my stomach on the wobbling ball. "I've got you. It's OK. Now lift your right leg up backward" *Ho yo.* Lucky rushed over and began licking my face. That was the last straw. In spite of Linda's best efforts I collapsed on the floor, convulsed with laughter. For the rest of the session we used the ball for more realistically designed exercises. I still have the ball and once in a while I practice some of the things I learned during that time. The ball is also great for the grandchildren until their mothers intervene when the play becomes too hectic. Some day we'll take it outdoors and we'll all have some real fun with it.

A big event in recovery was the day I drove the car again. Being driven around to one's various activities is all right at first. After all it's a joy to be able to join in things going on in the world after being confined, but it's also a restriction on one's autonomy not to be able to come and go without checking in with someone else's schedule. Everyone had been patient and helpful about chauffeuring me around but I did so want to be able to get myself around. I was beginning to understand the perspective of a two year old when he insists on doing everything himself. I remembered trying to help Brett get dressed when he was beginning to assert his independence and his cry of "Me do it, Grandma." Now this grandma wanted to me-do-it also.

I had practiced driving very short distances, to the end of the driveway and up to the garage again but I really felt liberated one day at the beginning of June, going on my own little expedition alone. *Would my legs work? Would my right ankle be strong enough for the brake pedal?*

*Would I remember how to drive?* All my fears were put to rest the day I drove away on my own like a baby bird leaving the nest.

# 22

## *Looking Back*

I will always remember those winter months when I could finally hoist myself up the stairs to have dinner with George in the kitchen. I treasured those meals cooked by "Chef George." After dinner I would spend the rest of the evening on the living room sofa in a contented blur. George had bought some classic movies on tape to augment our favorite television shows. For some reason I felt nurtured by the station break greeting used at the time by one of the national networks.

The smallest thing would make me teary. I lay in bed and reflected on the excellent nursing care I'd had in our city hospital. I remembered the discharge nurse and her concern for how I would be doing at home. I relived that moment on Christmas morning when I saw a star and felt in communion with God as a gentle peace settled over me like a soft blanket. I thought a lot about mortality, what I done with my life.

I had never done great deeds or accomplished big things; I was just plain old me with four children, five grandchildren and another one due in three months. I wanted to live long enough to let them all know how much they meant to me. I would say the names of George, my children and grandchildren, counting them off like precious pearls on a string. When it was time to purchase my traditional Valentines for all the children, I settled on writing each of them a note, telling what I found special about them and recalling some pleasant event. The project took several evenings and used a lot of my precious energy, but it was worth it. A psychologist might say that I was undergoing labile emotions brought on by trauma, but to me it felt good.

I had so much to be thankful for. Friends and family had showered George and me with kindness. There was a lot of food in the freezer—gifts of baked goods and bargains from George's forays into the world of grocery shopping. Our children had all kept track of my progress in the hospital. In fact, I heard that one medical student asked a nurse, "How many kids does that woman have, anyway?" It was my son who called me one morning in the hospital to inform me that I had a new student doctor that week. At times I think they knew more than I did about my condition. What made a big impression on me and on the nurses was the huge box of home made cookies my daughter-in-law sent. The night shift staff didn't leave many for the day shift.

We must have made quite a picture on those winter evenings: me stretched out on the sofa with a heating pad at my back and covered with a handmade afghan, George in one of our new reclining chairs, our big black sheepdog stretched out in the middle of the room. "We'll always remember this time in our lives," I murmured one evening.

George understood. "Yes," he said.

In early spring I began to keep a journal. On May 6th I wrote, *Such fatigue! Is this normal? Am I overdoing? Underdoing? What's right for this stage? Am I recovered? Should I push?* That time was almost more scary and frustrating than the time just before and after diagnosis. Then I was drugged and exhausted, sleeping away my days. But this was new territory and I had to face it all by myself. Many patients that I've talked to since have the same fear that plagued me at that time: Can this come back? Will I relapse? No caregiver can help a patient to come to a comfortable place in acceptance and adjustment during this phase of recovery.

The feeling of isolation was like being separated from the rest of humanity, unable to exchange information and ideas. One person whom I met face-to-face had suffered GBS in 1947 and been confined to an iron lung. I couldn't imagine anything so horrible. Moreover, paralysis had left her severely handicapped. Is this what will happen to me, I wondered. I would watch people out strolling with their dogs or walking briskly to get their heart rates up and tone their bodies and wonder if I would ever walk like that again. Then denial, my old friend, took up the burden for me and I was able to get through another day.

Denial can be a healthy thing if used judiciously and in small doses. It fends off needless worry. It enables a person to get through bad times, one day at a time. Tomorrow will be better, denial tells us. We'll just live through this one terrible moment and everything will be all right. A person in denial goes on automatic pilot and does what needs doing right at hand without thinking too far ahead. This state of mind is not to be confused with despair and depression, which can make a person shut down altogether. Healthy denial allows the individual to deal with adversity one step at a time without taking on too much at once.

Nonetheless, my journal shows some discouraging entries. *My walking is shaky and slow. My right leg continues to feel strange, like my skin is made of leather from the ankle down. And my big toe droops when I walk* Actually it felt like a tight rubber band was fastened around my right ankle. I still have to be careful to pick up my feet when I walk. When the myelin sheath began to repair itself and I felt the nerves coming back to life it was good to have assurance from the therapist that it was the "good pain." Never has something so good felt so bad. There are times even now when I feel discouraged: when I wake up in the morning with feet that are burning and tingling, when I tire easily and when I need to pace myself when working in my beloved garden. But then I stop and think of those days when I couldn't walk even with a walker or cane without tripping and I know how God has blessed me.

I returned to the classroom for the fall semester, still walking with a cane and limited to short distances, using my handicap placard in the parking lot. I felt like I had been in another world for the past nine months, but oh was it good to be back. My energy level was still way down and I would spend a couple of hours sleeping when I returned home every day. Never a big one for napping, naps were the name of the game in those days.

Still, I wished for some contact with former GBS patients. I had read the only two books I could find written for non medical people and we had found some stories on the Internet, but I longed to see a real live person who had emerged from the experience at least somewhat intact. Then one day a flyer arrived in the mail. Did George and I wish to drive down to the southern part of the state and attend a meeting for GBS patients and families. I lost no time in calling in our RSVP.

We were not disappointed; here was a whole family of GBS people. I'll never forget the feeling of wonder at being in the same room with so many other people who had had Guillain Barre. Seeing two of them in wheelchairs was my first realization that some people do not recover their former ways of life. That picture illustrates the cruelty of GBS and the capriciousness that governs who recovers and who does not. I heard a few horror stories from some of the people who looked completely recovered but who in fact were suffering hidden disabilities: legs that grow weak with use, bodies that fatigue easily. It was a humbling and enlightening experience.

That meeting and subsequent talks with the liaison there, drew me into the GBS community. Another Colorado liaison was needed for hospital visiting and increasing awareness of GBS in the northern part of the state. In my usual way of becoming involved, three years later I found myself standing at a podium before sixty people, introducing the speakers for our first Colorado GBS symposium. The flower that Jean had pinned to my lapel sent a sweet fragrance that mirrored my thoughts. I had learned to walk again on a different path.

# Epilogue

I have changed some of the names of medical personnel.

# APPENDIX

*Honest Medicine: Shattering the Myths About Aging and Health Care* by Donald J. Murphy, M.D. Atlantic Monthly Press: NY 1995

Dr. Murphy has served as medical director of the Senior Citizens Health Center at Presbyterian/St. Luke's Medical Center in Denver. He has also served as chairman of the Ethics Committee there.
This book explains how health care can be individually tailored with a bit of listening and common sense practice. Times are changing and seniors' attitudes of accepting doctors as the last word on what to do for healthy minds and bodies are changing as well. Doctors need no longer posture and patients need no longer passively accept. Health care, he says, is entering a new era and as the population of seniors grows, new approaches to individual needs must be taken. Also, we must debunk the myths of the one-size-fits-all strictures that the media has been laying out for us.

*Through the Patient's Eyes*
by Margaret Gerteis, et al., ed.
San Francisco: Jossey-Bass, 1993.

Technology is not enough in effective patient treatment. This book is the result of research that includes a national survey exploring hospital practices. Coordination of care and services, enhancing patients' physical comfort, providing emotional support, and involving family members are included in findings presented in this book.

*Bed Number Ten*
by Sue Baier 1985

This is a patient's account of Guillain Barre from the day of onset, the quick paralysis and the helpless state of dependence on others for the most basic human needs. Baier's experience with GBS included some health care professionals who were compassionate and empathic and some who could not imagine themselves in the patient's situation.

*Sick and Tired of Feeling Sick and Tired: Living with Invisible Chronic Illness*
by Paul J Donoghue, Ph.D and Mary E. Siegel, Ph.D., New York: Norton, 1992.

Pain and fatigue are hard to diagnose, hard to measure, and hard to live with This book acknowledges the frustration and humiliation suffered by people with all kinds of chronic illness. Included also is guidance on how to move forward with the best quality of life possible.

*Second Opinions: Stories of Intuition and Choice in the Changing World of Medicine*
by Jerome Groopman, M.D. New York: Viking 2000.

Dr. Groopman uses his own story and those of others to illustrate how we are ultimately the ones in charge of our well being. No medical decision is perfect. Fatigue, worry and pain, says Groopman often cloud our judgement. Patients and their families need to know when to question, when to search farther for answers and whom to trust.

*A Different Kind of Healing: Doctors Speak Candidly About their Successes with Alternative Medicine*
by Oscar Janiger, M.D. and Philip Goldberg.G.P.Putnam's Sons, NY,1993.

The premise of this book is that Western medicine, Eastern attitudes, and old fashioned natural remedies can work together in harmony to create an efficient, economical and facile health care system. However, homeopathic medicine should not be regarded as the end-all and be-all because some ailments do call for more aggressive and invasive treatment. Either camp—the conservatives and the progressives must avoid an elitist attitude toward the other. Above all, says Janiger, go with what the patient is comfortable with. This book is commonsense in its advice.

Guillain Barre Syndrome Foundation International web site:
**www.gbsfi.com**

Book Marketing Statement:
This book is for all Guillain Barre patients, their families and their physicians. It gives a human interest view of the disease and tells how one woman's life changed direction after recovery.

0-595-25823-9

Made in the USA
San Bernardino, CA
24 September 2016